OLDER PEOPLE AND
THE LAW

Ann McDonald and Margaret Tayl

D0533459

Consultant editor: Jo Campling

Revised Second Edition

First published as *Elders and the law* in 1993 by PEPAR Publications, Southside, 249 Ladypool Road, Birmingham, B12 8LF

This revised second edition published in Great Britain in November 2006 by

The Policy Press
University of Bristol
Fourth Floor
Beacon House
Queen's Road
Bristol BS8 1QU
UK

Tel +44 (0)117 331 4054
Fax +44 (0)117 331 4093
e-mail tpp-info@bristol.ac.uk
www.policypress.org.uk

© Ann McDonald and Margaret Taylor 2006

British Library Cataloguing in Publication Data
A catalogue record for this book is available from the British Library.

Library of Congress Cataloging-in-Publication Data
A catalog record for this book has been requested.

ISBN-10 1 86134 714 6 paperback
ISBN-13 978186134 714 5 paperback
ISBN-10 1 86134 715 4 hardcover
ISBN-13 978186134 715 2 hardcover

The right of Ann McDonald and Margaret Taylor to be identified as authors of this work has been asserted by them in accordance with the 1988 Copyright, Designs and Patents Act.

The statements and opinions contained within this publication are solely those of the author and not of The University of Bristol, The Policy Press or the British Association of Social Workers (BASW). The University of Bristol, The Policy Press and BASW disclaim responsibility for any injury to persons or property resulting from any material published in this publication.

The Policy Press works to counter discrimination on grounds of gender, race, disability, age and sexuality.

Cover design by Qube Design Associates, Bristol.
Front cover: photograph supplied by kind permission of Getty Images.
Printed and bound in Great Britain by Hobbs the Printers, Southampton.

Contents

Preface to the second edition v

Table of cases vii

Table of statutes, statutory instruments and treaties ... x

Introduction 1

one   **Social care in the community** 9
       Assessment 9
       Community care services provision 14
       Disability services 20
       Importance of the care plan 26
       Reviews 29
       Direct payments 30
       Carers' assessments and carers' services 33
       Abuse of older people 37
       Challenging decisions 43

two   **Health care needs** 53
       Legal basis of NHS care 54
       Responsibility for community health care 55
       Joint working 56
       NSF for older people 57
       Intermediate care 59
       NHS continuing care 60
       NHS treatment abroad 62
       Hospital discharge 63
       Palliative care 65
       Consent to treatment 66
       Mental incapacity 66
       End of life issues 70
       Mental health 73
       Challenging health care decisions 87

three **Housing and residential care** 91
       Housing 91
       Homelessness 94
       Entering residential care 96

four	**Financial management**	**111**
	Appointeeship	112
	Power of attorney	112
	Court of Protection – receivership	115
	Lifetime gifts	118
	Equity release schemes	118
	Undue influence	119
	Employment rights in older age	120
	Pensions	121
	Social security benefits	123
	Charging for non-residential services	131
	Paying for residential care	133
five	**Death and family provision**	**137**
	Funeral arrangements	137
	Coroners	138
	Distribution of estate	140
	Family provision	142
	Taxation	143
	Conclusion	147
	Appendix: List of organisations	149
	References	157
	Index	165

Preface to the second edition

The first edition of *Elders and the law* was published in 1993 in response to an identified gap for a brief, user-friendly book that brought together the various aspects of the law relating to older people. This is a topic of interest both to lawyers and to social workers and other professionals who have an interest in promoting the rights of older people and their access to health, social care and financial services. This may cover the whole range of services to support people in the community, through to admission to residential care and to hospital, and planning for end of life decisions, including the making of wills and dealing with the formalities of death. Few books cover this whole spectrum, and this book seeks in particular to link formal legal knowledge with an analysis of the social context in which law operates together with signposts to good practice. It is written by the original authors: a social work lecturer with a particular interest in community care, and a practising solicitor who deals with many older people and their families on a day-to-day basis. Opportunities for productive inter-professional working and dilemmas common to both professions are highlighted throughout the book, whose target audience is student social workers undertaking a qualifying degree programme. It is hoped, however, that the book will be of interest to other professionals, to older people themselves and to carers.

Demographic changes have led to an ageing population – the number of people over pensionable age in the UK is projected to increase from 11.4 million in 2006 to 12.2 million in 2011 and 15.2 million in 2031 (Age Concern, 2004). This will necessitate a re-appraisal of policies designed around the employment, financial and care needs of older people and of their individual aspirations. Social gerontology (Jamieson et al, 1997) requires us to look at ways in which age is constructed at a social level, particularly at institutions and practices that exclude or control older people. Professional groups also contribute to the creation of identities for older people as patients, or as service users, or clients. The development of community care policies and the growth of consumerism as well as changes in professional practice will therefore have an impact on the perceptions and experiences of older people.

Significant developments in health and social care, and in the legal framework that governs them, have taken place since 1993. For example, the first edition of this book looked forward to the implementation of the National Health Service (NHS) and Community Care Act 1990; that Act is now the central piece of legislation for the assessment of need for community care services. There have also been substantial reorganisations of the way in which services are delivered, particularly in the NHS, with the introduction of NHS trusts and the 'modernising' agenda leading to the development of a primary care-led NHS and, beyond this, an aspiration to a patient-led health care system (DH, 1997a). The *National service framework for older people* (DH, 2001a) concentrates on the needs of older people following strokes, falls and mental health problems, but also states the values of equal access to services and the promotion of active life expectancy. Such is the importance and complexity of changes within health care that a whole new chapter is devoted to them within this present edition. The introduction of direct payments and individual budgets instead of directly provided social care services also has the potential for transforming older people from recipients of care to active care managers employing personal assistants. Quality assurance in domiciliary as well as in residential care has been placed on a firmer national footing by the creation of national standards overseen by the Commission for Social Care Inspection (CSCI). National guidance on charging policies and the introduction of Pension Credit focuses attention on income maximisation. Considerable attention is given in this book to financial matters that affect older people, and ways of planning in advance for not being able to deal directly with finance oneself, and for organising inheritance and succession.

The change of title from *Elders and the law* for this second edition reflects current terminology in social work with older people. The book is divided into five chapters, covering social care in the community, health care, housing and residential care, finance and business affairs, and death and family provision. It highlights important areas of transition for older people, and opportunities for inter-professional working. Whereas the first edition did not explicitly relate the legal framework to the practice of social care with older people, this second edition contains a number of practice examples and case studies based on the application to practice of legal concepts and rules. A brief appendix gives details of where further advice and support can be found. There are suggestions for further reading at the end of each chapter.

Table of cases

Airedale NHS Trust v Bland [1993] 1 All ER 821   72
Aldridge and Hunt v Turner [2004] EWHC 2768 (Ch)   119
Alternative Futures case *see* R (Moore) v Care Standards Tribunal
An NHS Trust v M; An NHS Trust v H [2001] 2 FLR 367   72
An NHS Trust v X [2005] EWCA Civ 1145   71

B (Consent to Treatment: Capacity), Re [2002] All ER 429   73
Barrett v Enfield London Borough Council [2001] 2 AC 550   48, 95
Batantu v Islington London Borough Council [2000] All ER (D) 1744   95
Bolam v Friern Hospital [1957] 2 All ER 118   72, 87
Bournewood case *see* R v Bournewood Community and Mental Health NHS Trust
    ex parte L
Burke case *see* R (Burke) v GMC

Carty v Croydon London Borough Council [2005] EWCA Civ 19   48
Christopher Clunis v Camden and Islington Health Authority [1998] 3 All ER 180
    85
Coughlan case *see* R v North and East Devon Health Authority, ex parte Coughlan
Cunliffe v Fielden and another [2006] 2 All ER 115   143

F (Adult: Court's Jurisdiction), Re [2002] 3 WLR 1740   42-3

Gloucestershire case *see* R v Gloucestershire County Council ex parte Barry

Hammond v Osborn and another [2002] EWCA Civ 885   119-20
HL v UK (2004) 40 EHRR 761   80
HM v Switzerland (2002) Application 39187/98, European Court of Human Rights
    42

Jones v Manchester Corporation [1952] 2 All ER 125   87
JT v UK [2000] 1 FLR 909   76-7

K, Re [1988] 2 FLR 15   113

McCann v UK (1998) 28 EHRR 245   139
Masterman-Lister v Brutton and Co; Masterman-Lister v Jewell and another [2003] 3
    All ER 162   115-16

North Devon Homes v Brazier [2003] EWHC 574   93

Portsmouth NHS Trust v Wyatt [2004] EWHC 2247   71
Pretty v DPP [2002] 1 All ER 1   73
Pretty v UK [2002] 2 FCR 97   73

R (A & B) v East Sussex County Council and another (no 1) [2003] EWHC 167 (Admin)   132

R (B) v Camden London Borough Council [2005] EWHC 1366 (Admin)   19

R (Beeson) v Dorset County Council [2002] EWCA Civ 1812   134

R (Burke) v General Medical Council [2005] EWCA Civ 1003   72-3

R (Calgin) v Enfield London Borough Council [2005] EWHC 1716   96

R (D) v Haringey London Borough Council [2005] EWHC 2235 (Admin)   56, 87

R (Dudley and Whitbread and others) v East Sussex County Council [2003] EWHC 1093 Admin   102-3

R (Goldsmith) v Wandsworth London Borough Council [2004] EWCA Civ 1170   65

R (Grogan) v Bexley NHS Care Trust [2006] EWHC 44 (Admin)   61

R (Gunter) v Southwest Staffordshire PCT [2005] EWHC 1894 (Admin)   65

R (H) v Secretary of State for Health [2005] All ER (D) 218   83

R (H) v Secretary of State for the Home Department and others [2003] 3 WLR 1278   48

R (on the application of Heather and others) v The Leonard Cheshire Foundation and the Attorney General [2002] All ER 936   103

R (Hooper) v Secretary of State for Work and Pensions [2006] 1 All ER 487   126

R (HP and KP) v Islington London Borough Council [2004] EWHC 7 (Admin)   74

R (K) v West London Mental Health NHS Trust [2006] EWCA Civ 118   80-1

R (Moore) v Care Standards Tribunal [2005] 1 WLR 2979   103

R (on the application of E) v Bristol City Council [2005] All ER (D) 57   77

R (on the application of Goodson) v Bedfordshire and Luton Coroner [2004] EWHC 2931   140

R (on the application of Gunter) v South Western Staffordshire PCT [2005] EWHC 1894   132

R (on the application of Mari) v Lambeth London Borough Council [2003] EWCA Civ 836   17

R (on the application of SSG) v Liverpool City Council and Secretary of State for Health (CO/1220/2002)   77

R (on the application of Takoushis) v Inner London North Coroner and another [2005] EWCA Civ 1440   140

R (on the application of Westminster City Council) v NASS [2002] 1 WLR 2956   98

R (Stephenson) v Stockton-on-Tees Borough Council [2005] WLR (D) 102   36

R v Ashworth Hospital Authority ex parte Munjaz [2005] UKHL 58   75

R v Avon CC, ex parte M [1994] 2 FLR 1006   44

R v Avon County Council, ex parte M [1994] 2 FCR 259   100-1

R v Birmingham City Council, ex parte Killigrew (2000) 3 CCLR 109   28-9

R v Birmingham City Council ex parte Taj Mohammed (1998) 1 CCLR 441   25

R v Bournewood Community and Mental Health NHS Trust ex parte L [1999] 1 WLR 107   79-80, 86

R v Bristol City London Borough Council ex parte Penfold (1998) 1 CCLR 315   11, 97

R v Cumbria County Council ex parte Cumbria Professional Care Ltd (2000) 3 CCLR 79   102

R v Gloucestershire County Council ex parte Barry [1997] AC 584   23, 28, 29, 48, 98

R v HM Coroner for the County of West Yorkshire ex parte Sacker and R v HM Coroner for the Western District of Somerset, ex parte Middleton [2004] All ER (D) 268   139

R v Islington London Borough Council ex parte Rixon (1998) 1 CCLR 119   26

R v Kensington and Chelsea London Borough Council ex parte Kujtim 28 [1999] 4 All ER 161   28

R v Kirklees Metropolitan Borough Council ex parte Daykin (1998) 1 CCLR 512   25

R v Lanarkshire County Council ex parte McGregor (2000) 4 CCLR 188   99-100

R v Manchester County Council ex parte Stennett and others [2002] 3 WLR 584   83, 84, 85

R v North and East Devon Health Authority, ex parte Coughlan [2000] 1 WLR 622   55, 56, 60, 61, 102

R v Richmond London Borough Council and others ex parte Watson [2001] 1 All ER 436   84

R v Secretary of State for Social Services, ex parte West Midlands Health Authority and Birmingham Area Health Authority, ex parte Hincks [1980] 1 BMLR 93   54

R v Sefton Metropolitan Borough Council ex parte Help the Aged [1997] All ER 532   98

R v Waltham Forest London Borough Council ex parte Vale (1985) *The Times*, 25 February   96

R v Wandsworth London Borough Council, ex parte Beckwith [1996] All ER 129   99

R v Westminster City Council ex parte P and others (1998) 1 CCLR 486   46

R (Wahid) v Tower Hamlets London Borough Council [2002] EWCA Civ 287   97

R (Watts) v Bedford PCT [2006] All ER (D) 220 (May)   62

Richards v Secretary of State for Works and Pensions (Case C-423/04, 2006)   122

S (Hospital Patient: Court's Jurisdiction), Re [1996] Fam 1   42

Sefton case *see* R v Sefton Metropolitan Borough Council ex parte Help the Aged

Shah v London Borough of Barnet [1983] 2 AC 309   96

Sidaway v Bethlem Royal Hospital Governors [1985] 1 All ER 643   66

Stennett case *see* R v Manchester County Council ex parte Stennett and others

W and others v Essex County Council and another [2000] 2 All ER 237   48

W v Egdell [1990] 1 All ER 835   14

Watts case *see* R (Watts) v Bedford PCT

Westminster London Borough Council v NASS [2002] 1 WLR 2956   17

Wyatt v Hillingdon London Borough Council [1978] 76 LGR 727   46

X (Minors) v Bedfordshire County Council [1995] All ER 353   49

Z (Local Authority: Duty), Re [2005] 1 WLR 959   73

Z and others v UK (2002) 34 EHRR 3   49

Table of statutes, statutory instruments and treaties

Statutes

Administration of Estates Act 1925   142

Care Standards Act 2000   45, 104, 107
  s 1   105
  s 3   105
  s 13(3)   106
  s 14   108
  s 20   108
  s 23   107
  s 24   106
  s 121(1)   105
  s 121(9)   105
Carers and Disabled Children Act 2000   30, 34–5
  s 2   37
  s 2(3)   37
Carers (Equal Opportunities) Act 2004   35
Carers (Recognition and Services) Act 1995   34
Children Act 1989   1, 42
  s 47   38
Chronically Sick and Disabled Persons Act 1970   16, 18, 20
  s 1   21
  s 2   14, 18, 19, 22–3, 26, 46, 48, 56
Civil Partnership Act 2004   86, 122
Community Care (Delayed Discharges) Act 2003   35, 63–4, 97
  s 4(2)   64
  s 5   64
Community Care (Direct Payments) Act 1996   30
Coroners Act 1988   138
  s 8(3)(d)   139
Crime and Disorder Act 1998   39

Data Protection Act 1998   13–14
Disability Discrimination Act 1995   20, 93
  ss 13, 16   93–4

Disabled Persons (Services, Consultation and Representation) Act 1986   20
  s 4   21, 22
  s 9   21
Domestic Violence, Crime and Victims Act 2004   39
  s 6   39

Employment Relations Act 1999   36
Enduring Powers of Attorney Act 1985   113
Environmental Protection Act 1990   42
Equality Act 2006   121

Family Law Act 1996, Part IV   39
Freedom of Information Act 2000, s 19   14

Health Act 1999   24
  s 27   53
  s 31   53
Health and Social Care Act 2001
  Part III   53
  s 49   55–6
  ss 53–55   133
  s 53   98, 101
  ss 57, 58   30
Health and Social Care (Community Health and Standards) Act 2003   45, 88, 104
Health and Social Services and Social Security Adjudications Act 1983
  s 17   26, 131
  s 21   134
  s 22   134
Health Services and Public Health Act 1968   16
  s 45   17, 18, 19
Homelessness Act 2002   95
Housing Act 1985, Schedule 5, para 11   92–3
Housing Act 1996   95
  Part VII   94

s 193   94–5
Housing Grants, Construction and
    Regeneration Act 1996   24
    Part 1   24
    s 23   24–5
    s 24(3)   25
    s 34   26
Human Rights Act 1998   5, 7, 42, 47,
    50, 64, 72, 82, 102, 103, 147
    s 7   5, 50
Human Tissues Act 2004   138–9

Immigration and Asylum Act 1999, s 115
    17
Inheritance (Provision for Family and
    Dependants) Act 1975   142, 143

Local Authority Social Services Act
    1970   3
    s 7   4, 43
    s 7D   46
Local Government Act 2000   47
Local Government and Housing Act
    1989, s 5   47

Medicines Act 1968   106
Mental Capacity Act 2005   43, 66, 73,
    86, 112, 113, 114, 117
    s 1   66
    s 2   67
    s 3   67
    s 4   69, 70
    s 5   69–70
    s 9   67, 69
    s 15   67
    ss 24–26   68
    s 24   67
    s 25(4)(c)   68–9
    s 35   67–8
    s 39   99
    s 40   67
    s 44   40
Mental Health Act 1959   81
Mental Health Act 1983   4, 31, 41, 42,
    48, 74, 75–6, 79–80, 85, 107, 140
    s 1(2)   77
    s 1(3)   77
    s 2   77, 78, 83
    s 3   77, 78–9, 83, 84

s 4   78
s 7(1)   81
s 8(2)   81
s 12   76
s 17   80
s 22   77
s 26   76–7
s 26(6)   77
s 29   77
s 37   83
ss 47, 48   83
s 72   82–3
ss 93–113   115
s 94(2)   113
s 115   79
s 117   16, 19–20, 48, 83–4, 85, 99,
    131, 134
s 129   79
s 131   76
s 135   79
s 136   79
s 139   48

National Assistance Act 1948   99
    Part III   16
    s 21   16–17, 20, 60, 83, 95, 96, 97–
        8, 102, 108
    s 21(1)(c)   96, 97
    s 21(1A)   17
    s 21(2A)   98
    s 22   133
    s 26(3A)   102
    s 28A   96
    s 29   16, 17, 19, 20–1, 24
    s 47   41
National Assistance (Amendment) Act
    1951   41
National Health Service Act 1977   3,
    19, 54, 55, 56, 57, 60
    s 1(1)   54
    s 21   16, 17
    Schedule 5A   132
    Schedule 8   16
    Schedule 8, para 3(1)   18
National   Health   Service   and
    Community Care Act 1990   v, 4,
    10, 11, 34
    s 42(2)   104
    s 46(3)   16, 37, 83

s 47   12, 14, 41, 42, 63, 74, 84
s 47(1)   9–10
s 47(1)(b)   14, 26
s 47(2)   14, 21-2
s 47(3)(a)   56
s 50   43

Powers of Attorney Act 1971, s 10   112
Prevention of Eviction Act 1977   92
Protection from Harassment Act 1997
    40
    s 5   40
Public Health (Control of Disease) Act
    1984   137

Registered Homes Act 1984   104, 105
    s 5(3)   106

Social Security Contributions and
    Benefits Act 1992, s 73   131

Unfair Contract Terms Act 1977, s 2
    102

Welfare Reform and Benefits Act 1999
    126
Wills Act 1837   141

Youth Justice and Criminal Evidence Act
    1999, Part II 40

Statutory instruments
Care Homes Regulations 2001 (SI
    2001/3965)   107
    reg 4   107–8
    reg 14   108
    reg 15   108
    reg 23   107
    Schedule 1   108
Commission for Social Care Inspection
    (Fees and Frequency of Inspection)
    (Amendment) Regulations 2006 (SI
    2006/517)   108
Community Care, Services for Carers
    and Children's Services (Direct
    Payments) (England) Regulations
    2003 (SI 2003/762)   30–1
    reg 2(1)(a)   31
    reg 6   31

Coroners Rules 1984 (SI 1984/552)
    138
Court of Protection (Enduring Powers
    of Attorney) Rules 2001 (SI 2001/
    825)   113

Employment Equality (Age)
    Regulations 2006 (SI 2006/1031)
    120-1

National Health Service (General
    Medical Services) Regulations 1992
    (SI 1992/635)   57

Treaties
European Community Treaty, Article 49
    62
European Convention on Human Rights
    5, 7, 75, 76, 82, 86
    Article 2   72, 102, 103, 139, 140
    Article 3   49, 72, 102
    Article 5   80, 83
    Article 6   44
    Article 8   64-5, 72, 77, 95, 102
    Article 13   49

Introduction

Older people are not an homogeneous group and their needs are diverse. As a concept, old age is socially constructed according to the expectations of society, and the social roles that are ascribed to older people may not correlate with their own views of their wishes and needs. At one end of the spectrum, some leisure services are available for those aged 50 plus; financial services may correlate with 'pensionable' age (currently 60 for women and 65 for men); and some services, for example health care checks, may be focused on the over-75s according to their physical vulnerability. This means that planning and providing services for older people has to cover a range of ages that may span two generations. Some older people will be survivors of a generation born at the beginning of the last century, and others will be post-war baby boomers. This 'cohort' effect of having lived through different periods of social change may mean that their expectations of family life, of the role of the state and of acceptable standards of living, are different. Individually also, their different experiences across the lifecourse will have shaped the people that they become (Hockey and James, 2003). It is not uncommon for 'younger' older people to take responsibility for the care of their parent as an 'older' older person, a situation for which there is no cultural precedent and which was unrecognised legally until the recent introduction of legislation on carers. Older people will therefore experience ageing differently based on their personal history as well as their gender, class, 'race' and culture. They may, because of their social position or personal situation, be more or less able to be proactive in securing whatever legal rights are available to them, and will need varying degrees of support to do so.

Absence of a legal framework relating solely to older people

In any case there is no single body of law relating specifically to older people, which distinguishes them as people with individual or collective rights. This can be compared with the position of children for whom the Children Act 1989 operates as a unifying piece of legislation. Older people are, on the whole, not distinguished in a legal sense from any other group of adults. Their capacity to make decisions about their own welfare is assumed, and other family members have no automatic legal duties towards them. The state's responsibility to provide services for health and social care is based not on age but on the presence of a disability or mental health issue, and proactive intervention is not based on a particular status being given to old age, but on the general law. It may be argued that this absence of a distinct legal status for old age protects the citizenship of older people and prevents their adult status being undermined in a paternalistic way. But it does mean that it is difficult to establish an agreed value base for decision making at critical times for older people, particularly at the end of life. It also means that the role of family members or other carers is unclear. But most importantly from a legal perspective, it means that giving advice to older people requires the pulling together of information from a wide range of disparate sources, often amending concepts developed for use in other situations.

Older people themselves may also have different views of the law. Their particular views are likely to reflect previous experience. Some may see the law as something to be feared and avoided, if they think predominantly in terms of criminal law; others may see the law as a way of putting their affairs in order, if they have used the law to make a will or to invest in property. People generally will recognise that the law gives rights and imposes duties. They may also use the law to deal with grievances and to seek remedies. In this, they may be confident that the law will be fair and impartial, or they may see the law as weighted in favour of property owners or officialdom. When scarce resources have to be rationed, the law will be used to decide who gets how much of what type of benefit. Having a fair process to make decisions is another function of the law. The law may also regulate private organisations for the public good, so, for example, private providers of residential care are highly regulated by an inspection regime that is based on detailed rules and common standards.

Professional roles

In order to use the law, affected individuals and groups will need to have access to legal advice. This may mean that they approach a legal adviser directly or seek information from a statutory or voluntary organisation that can explain their legal position and help them to act on it. In this way, the social worker may be seen as a person who should be competent in knowing about the law. Social workers are experienced in working with a range of other professionals, but these are usually from the health professions; direct inter-professional working with lawyers is less common. Similarly, lawyers may have only occasional contact with social workers, meaning that each profession may have to make some effort to learn the other's language or style of working. They may also need to clarify their different allegiances – where the lawyer's role is directly to act as an advocate for the client, presenting their point of view, the social worker may have to balance the needs of the client against those of other family members, or of the public, or of their own organisation.

Whereas in private practice the solicitor's client is the older person, when social workers need to make decisions they themselves may become the client seeking legal advice. In reality of course there is considerable ambiguity within the traditional formula 'the lawyer advises, the client instructs', and lawyers may become more directly involved in what they see as 'social work' advice and decision making (Dickens, 2004). For the social worker, their professional obligations are set out in the *Code of practice for social care workers* (GSCC, 2002). For the lawyer, their professional duties are set out in the Law Society's *Guide to the professional conduct of solicitors* (Law Society, 1999). The first question to be asked by the lawyer is: who is my client? This may not be the relative, carer or neighbour who makes the first approach. After that, instructions need to be taken from the client (preferably seeing them alone at least once) and given free of another's influence, checks made that the client has the requisite capacity and any potential conflict of interest identified early on so that independent legal advice can be recommended for third parties where need be.

Sources of law

The basic starting point in the application of law to practice is the ability to recognise the pervasiveness of legal issues (Ball and McDonald, 2003). There are a number of different sources of law that define the rights and duties both of agencies and individuals. Agencies such as social services authorities and NHS trusts are statutory bodies, the powers of which are derived from legislation. For the social services authorities the founding statute is the Local Authority Social Services Act 1970, while most health care powers and duties can be traced back to the National Health Service (NHS) Act 1977. Increasingly, the operation of statute law cannot be understood from a reading of the Act alone; the detailed legal rules are contained in statutory instruments – rules and regulations for administrative decision making. In giving directions to local authorities on the proper interpretation of their legal powers, the Secretary of State for Health may seek uniformity in decision making on an administrative level. An example of this is the Community Care Assessment Directions 2004 that require local authorities actively to involve potential service users and carers in assessments. In addition, the Secretary of State may issue guidance to local authorities on policies that they wish to see implemented. If this is 'Section (s) 7 guidance', this is a reference to s 7 of the Local Authority Social Services Act 1970 that requires local authorities to 'act under' the general guidance of the Secretary of State. Local authorities may depart from such guidance only if they can produce specific reasons for doing so, and even then they cannot follow a substantially different route. The policy guidance *Community care in the next decade and beyond* (DH, 1990), which describes the care management process, is such s 7 guidance. Beyond this, local authorities also have to 'take into account' practice guidance on how such policy should be implemented, and an example of this is the important practitioners' guide to the NHS and Community Care Act 1990 (DH, 1991a). There is thus a complex hierarchy of material that needs to be assimilated into any decision-making process carried out by a statutory agency. It is also important to bear in mind throughout the distinction between powers and duties – services that the local authority may provide and those that it must provide.

There are many areas of activity that are governed not by statute law, but by the common law – by the body of law that has been developed by the courts into a network of legal principles. Much of the law of contract is common law, as is the law of tort, covering civil wrongs such as negligence, trespass and defamation. Common law develops on a case-by-case basis where decided cases clarify legal principles. But statute law also has to be interpreted, so that, to understand how the law is applied, it is necessary in this book to look at examples of case law. This is particularly important when trying to predict how contested terms such as 'reasonable', 'adequate' and 'substantial' may be interpreted. When people are in competition for scarce resources, such interpretations may be helpful in arguing for the legitimacy of a claim. There are also areas where common law concepts such as 'incapacity' have to be interpreted. Even the term 'mental illness' used within the Mental Health Act 1983 is not defined in statute, but through usage sanctioned by the courts. Getting access to the legal system as an important source of authority for making cases into precedents is crucial therefore to the development of the law. In some cases, the law has been moved forward by critical 'test cases', sometimes brought by organisations with an interest in achieving clarity in the law. Help the Aged and RADAR have helped individuals to take action in this way.

The most significant recent legal development, however, has been the enactment of the Human Rights Act 1998, which has brought the major provisions of the European Convention on Human Rights directly into English law (Watson and Woolf, 2003). Some of the Articles of the European Convention on Human Rights may be of direct relevance to older people – for example, Article 2, the right to life; Article 3, the right to freedom from inhuman or degrading treatment; Article 8, the right to privacy and family life; and Article 14, the prohibition on discrimination in the enjoyment of the other rights and freedoms granted by the Convention. In addition, under s 7 of the Human Rights Act 1998 there is a right of action against public authorities for breaches of Convention rights, and modest awards of compensation are possible.

Social policy context

This is the legal framework within which issues chosen for their direct relevance to older people will be discussed in this book. The current social policy context is still heavily influenced by ideas developed when the system of community care was introduced in the early 1990s, by the Thatcher government. The impetus behind the development of community care has been well documented elsewhere (McDonald, 2006), but three fundamental influences can be discerned: political ideas of personal responsibility and choice; the development of a mixed economy of care; and the rise of care management as a method of social work intervention. The 'modernising' work of New Labour continues to emphasise equality of opportunity rather than rights to services, although with a greater emphasis on central control over standards (for example, through national service frameworks in health care) and the creation of new regulatory bodies to monitor quality both in the public and in the independent sector. One change, however, has been the replacement of competition with the idea of partnership. Legalism in the sense of generating and applying formal rules for decision making has been a continuing feature of the community care system, determining criteria for carrying out assessments, for targeting services and for paying for services. Legalism has also supported consumerism in specifying minimum standards of care to which 'service users' are entitled, and providing new means of redress for their breach through complaints procedures and legal actions. A legal lens through which social workers can view their role with older people is particularly appropriate therefore in the community care context.

The emphasis on personal responsibility in planning for ageing is also seen in the benefits and pensions system. The general move from benefits to tax credits does not seek to penalise people who have modest savings, and rewards prudence in planning for retirement. Demographic changes have meant that the state pensions system will no longer be adequate on its own to support a reasonable standard of living in retirement. The emphasis then is on personal pension planning alongside occupational pensions for people in employment. Family expectations that they will inherit money and property will also have to be managed in this changed context. Social workers also will be influenced in their practice by a political agenda that emphasises competition and self-reliance, and judged on their performance according to national as well as local performance indicators.

The modernising agenda in health and social care (DH, 1997a, 1998a) has moved debates on from welfare provision to 'well-being' (DH, 2004a). The Green Paper on adult social care (DH, 2005a) envisages individuals having greater choice over services and more personal responsibility for managing their own health and necessary care services. There is a greater emphasis on prevention and 'inverting the triangle of care' (ADSS, 2003) so that people with lower level needs receive more support to remain in the community. Older people themselves (Clark et al, 2004; Walker, 2005) value low-level services that are preventative and community based, but also see their involvement in the planning and prioritising of services as a necessary part of citizenship. The White Paper on adult health and social care (DH, 2006a) takes further this preventative agenda, and will set the agenda for the development of health and social care services for the next decade. The whole question of the proper balance between public funding and individual responsibility for paying for care services has been opened up again for debate by the Wanless report (2006), which brings together economic, ethical and political debate about the role of the state.

Discrimination against older people

Services for older people may in their design or in their delivery be influenced by ageism and by discrimination (Norman, 1985). Help the Aged defines ageism as "prejudging or making assumptions about people simply because of their age" (Help the Aged, 2002). Age discrimination is the institutionalisation of that prejudice in policy or custom and practice. A survey for the King's Fund (Roberts, 2000) found that three out of four senior managers working in health and social services believed that age discrimination occurred within local services. The Human Rights Act 1998 prohibits discrimination in the enjoyment of rights guaranteed by the European Convention. European Community law also prohibits discrimination on the basis of age, although this is restricted to employment matters. It has been used successfully to challenge different retirement (although not pensionable) ages for men and women even though this was not provided for in national legislation. The Equal Treatment Directive (2000) requires member states to introduce legislation to outlaw discrimination in employment by 2006. The relationship between legal change and changing attitudes will need to be monitored at a cultural as well as at an individual level. Research conducted for Age Concern (Age Concern/University of Kent, 2005) found that more people reported suffering age discrimination than any other form of discrimination, while one in three respondents said they viewed the over-70s as incompetent and incapable. These findings present a clear challenge for legislators and for the value base of social work practice and legal decision making. Raising as it does an insight into the inter-relationship between different types of discrimination, this discussion of ageism is a direct challenge to anti-discriminatory practice with older people.

Social work role

The social work role with older people will therefore need to incorporate dealing with the impact of discrimination, into a therapeutic or professional relationship. At the same time, economic imperatives behind the rationing of resources will require individual practitioners to facilitate such things as rapid discharge from hospital or cuts in community care services, which disproportionately affect older people. A professional dissonance is therefore created between the 'idea' of community care and its reality (Postle, 2002).

The requirements for social work training at qualifying level provide an agenda that is easily translatable to the main tasks within social work for older people. *National occupational standards* (TOPSS, 2001) describe social work in terms of key roles:

Key role 1:   Prepare for and work with individuals, families, carers, groups and communities to assess their needs and circumstances.

Key role 2:   Plan, carry out, review and evaluate social work practice with individuals, families, carers, groups and communities and other professionals.

Key role 3:   Support individuals to represent their needs, views and circumstances.

Key role 4:   Manage risk to individuals, families, carers, groups, communities, self and colleagues.

Key role 5:   Manage and be accountable, with supervision and support, for your own social work practice within your organisation.

Key role 6:   Demonstrate professional competence in social work practice.

Each of these key roles incorporates legal issues that will be examined within the following chapters. Social work as a combination of knowledge, skills and values mirrors the attributes of law insofar as legal knowledge by itself does not answer professional dilemmas. Working with vulnerable people requires skills in eliciting information, conveying knowledge and balancing risks. It also requires a strong value base of showing respect for the integrity of individuals and valuing their history and strengths that is particularly important with older people.

Having confidence in their knowledge of the law and being able to cite legal arguments to support their case and to challenge others' decisions are key skills for social workers' training (Braye and Preston-Shoot, 2005). Service users will also expect social workers to possess and to be able to apply legal knowledge in their practice. Hence the 'Statement of expectations', which is an appendix to the *National occupational standards for social workers*, emphasises the following: social workers must explain their role and the purpose of contact and their powers, *including their legal powers*; social workers should be able to challenge their organisation on behalf of service users and carers and challenge poor practice; and social workers should possess knowledge of relevant services provided by other organisations, and knowledge of welfare benefits and relevant legislation. There is a considerable agenda therefore for social workers to meet in terms of legal skills and knowledge. This combination of being the holder of legal duties, of being able to distinguish duties from powers where there is discretion, being able to acknowledge older people's rights as citizens and as service users, and providing effective remedies where rights are denied, is central to the professional role of the social worker (Preston-Shoot, 2000), and exactly reflects the structure and language of legal argument.

ONE

Social care in the community

The traditional view of the welfare state, based on the idea of social unity and social justice, viewed older people as a cohesive but dependent group. The developing concept of the 'enabling' state that was the basis of community care policy replaced state provision with a consumerist view of citizenship within which there was competition between different groups for scarce resources. Higgs (1997) relates this changing view of citizenship to the position of older people and the nature of legal rights. He points out the contradictory nature of citizenship based on choice for older people, where the most frail cannot exercise choice as consumers. He also sees a move away from collective substantive rights for older people as a group, towards procedural rights for individuals. The provision of community care services is a good example of such consumerism in action as services such as domiciliary care and residential care previously provided directly by local authorities have become privatised and tightly rationed. But Higgs (1997) also sees a third stage, a move from rights to surveillance, with the monitoring of deviation from an ideal of competent old age based on notions of risk to self and to the community.

For people with more complex needs, the gateway to a 'mixed economy of care' of public and private sector resources is through an assessment by professionals, increasingly with an emphasis on risk avoidance and protection. When resources are scarce, access to a procedurally correct assessment of need assumes greater importance, and it is the legal requirements of assessment, care planning and review within a system of care management but also as key social work tasks that will be looked at in this chapter.

Assessment

Assessment, however, is not only the gateway to the provision of community care services; it can also be a service in its own right, making people aware of services that are available and helping them to make choices between different options. The legal duty to assess is contained in s 47(1) of the NHS and Community Care Act 1990, which says that:

Where it appears to a local authority that any person for whom they may provide or arrange for the provision of community care services may be in need of any such services, the authority –

(a)   shall carry out an assessment of his needs for those services; and

(b)   having regard to the results of that assessment shall then decide whether his needs call for the provision by them of any such services.

It is worth noting that (a) and (b) are conceptually distinct; the assessment of a need for services is separate from the decision whether or not services should be provided. It is the *appearance* of need that triggers the duty to assess, not a request for a service. Of course, few people ask for 'an assessment of need'; most enquire about their eligibility for a particular service such as home care or residential care. But the statutory duty is to assess the person's need for any of a range of services, and only then to make a decision on which services will be provided. The 'trigger' questions that the frontline worker has to ask within a screening assessment should at a minimum identify the complexity of the situation and should explore the services that the person receives from other agencies, any carers' issues and the urgency of the need. An assessment may be of future needs, for example, on discharge from hospital, but although assessment is 'needs-led', it is not, from a legal perspective, 'user-led', because, as we will see, it is the local authority that determines what 'needs' are, as well as how they will be met.

Local authorities carrying out needs assessments will do so within a framework laid down by the Secretary of State for Health. For older people, this will be:

* *Care management and assessment: Practitioners' guide* (DH, 1991a) (the practice guidance under the NHS and Community Care Act 1990);
* *Fair access to care services: Guidance on eligibility criteria for adult social care* (DH, 2002a);
* *National service framework for older people* (DH, 2001a) and the detailed guidance on *The single assessment* process (DH, 2002b). This is more fully discussed on page 12;
* *Directions on the carrying out of the assessment process to ensure the involvement of potential service users and carers* (DH, 2004b).

It is the responsibility of the social worker to guide the way through the assessment process. Practice guidance under the NHS and Community Care Act 1990 (DH, 1991a) adopts a due process model insofar as practitioners must ensure that users understand:

- what is involved in the assessment procedures;
- the likely timescale;
- what authority the practitioner holds;
- their entitlement to information, participation and representation. (DH, 1991a, para 3.16)

When resources are scarce, it is important to be clear about the definition of 'need' and its source: is it need as defined by older people themselves, or by the assessor? The *Practitioners' guide* (DH, 1991a, para 11) defines needs as "the requirements of individuals to enable them to achieve, maintain or restore an acceptable level of social independence or quality of life, as defined by the particular care agency or authority". Translating assessed need into service provision is mediated by the eligibility criteria specifying who is to receive a service based on level of need and/or risk. Presenting needs are relevant to the assessment process insofar as they reflect the accounts that individuals give of their own needs for service. Importantly, the fair access to care services guidance on eligibility (DH, 2002a) (see below) restates the judgment in the *Penfold* case [1998] 1 CCLR 315, that the threshold for assessment of presenting needs is 'low'. Paragraph 30 of *Fair access to care services* (DH, 2002a) makes it clear that local authorities should not operate eligibility criteria for the type and depth of assessment that they carry out and should not screen individuals out of the assessment process before sufficient information is known about them. So, on the facts of the *Penfold* case, Mrs Penfold, who had a history of anxiety and depression and who had moved to the area to be closer to relatives, was entitled to an assessment although there were limited prospects of someone with such low-level needs being given a service by the local authority. Any assessment carried out by the local authority in the area from which the applicant has moved will also be a relevant consideration to take into account. The important point is that assessment issues precede any decisions on eligibility for services, and that the assessment duty is an individual one, not simply a way of fitting people into available services. Legal duty and good practice in promoting an exchange model of assessment (Smale and Tuson, 1993) therefore coalesce at this point.

Assessment directions

The community care assessment directions 2004 (DH, 2004b) similarly place existing good practice on conducting assessments and care planning into a legal framework. Paragraph 2 of the directions says that when assessing the needs of a person under s 47 of the NHS and Community Care Act 1990 the local authority must:

- consult the person, consider whether the person has any carers and, where they think it appropriate, consult those carers (para 2.2);
- take all reasonable steps to reach agreement with the person and any carers on community care services which they are considering providing to him to meet his needs (para 2.3);
- provide information about the amount of payment for which the person will be liable (para 2.4).

The directions clarify that when the assessment is of an older person, the requirements of the Single Assessment Process (SAP) should be observed, and that assessments for all adults with complex needs should take account of physical, cognitive, behavioural and social participation needs (DH, 2002b, para 2.5). Where it is inappropriate to involve the carer, the local authority should retain a written account of the reasons for this. The directions thus require local authorities to incorporate partnership principles into care management systems, and to maximise opportunities for information sharing.

Single Assessment Process for older people

Guidance on SAP (DH, 2002b) is designed to promote person-centred care within integrated assessment, commissioning and care planning arrangements. Whatever the professional background of the assessor, SAP enables an holistic assessment to begin by identifying information needs that become progressively more complex. So all users/patients will have a 'contact assessment' where basic personal information is collected and the nature of the presenting problem is explored to establish the presence of wider health and/or social care issues. This may then lead to an 'overview assessment', still carried out by a trained and competent single professional, looking at a wide range of needs. The overview assessment may indicate a need for specialist assessment to focus on a specific need, for example for assistive technology, or specialist equipment or adaptations. A 'comprehensive assessment' covers all or most of the domains of need (see below) and will involve a range of professionals or specialist teams. Such an assessment will take place where the level of support or treatment indicated is likely to be intensive or prolonged, such as an intensive package of care at home or discharge from hospital to intermediate care. In social work terms, SAP is a tool for facilitating 'case finding' by agencies; it supports classic models of social work intervention that are task-centred, systems-based and crisis-responsive (Lymbery, 2005).

There are a number of validated 'tools' available to carry out assessments under SAP, although Cornes and Clough (2004) identify that most of them are based on medical rather than social models of diagnosis and treatment. The structure of SAP is built on nine areas or 'domains' of need that impact on the older person's independence, health and recovery and rehabilitation. These domains are:

- user's perspective
- clinical background
- disease prevention
- personal care and physical well-being
- senses
- mental health
- relationships
- safety
- immediate environment and resources.

The primary purpose of SAP is to prevent procedures being needlessly duplicated by different agencies. Case information on an individual older person is stored and shared, subject to consent and confidentiality, among health and social care professionals, through the development of a 'current summary record'. Information sharing protocols have also been devised as route maps for implementing information sharing policies. The Centre for Policy on Ageing (see the Appendix) is acting as a repository for professional learning and development materials based on SAP.

Freedom of information and confidentiality

The most important source of the duty to keep information confidential is the Data Protection Act 1998. The Act applies to paper records and computer-held data and covers any information or personal data that relates to an identifiable individual. Commonly service users are asked to give written consent to the disclosure of confidential information to other agencies in the course of a community care assessment. Such consent may be implied where necessary to provide proper care; this would include disclosure to service providers. In other cases, the public interest can override confidentiality to create a duty of disclosure on professionals, as in *W v Egdell* [1990] 1 All ER 835, where a psychiatrist who had compiled a report for a mental health review tribunal at the request of the patient's solicitor was under a duty to disclose its content to the tribunal and the Home Office, although it was adverse to the patient. Section 19 of the Freedom of Information Act 2000 requires public authorities to list the information, for example policies and procedures, that the organisation has in its possession. This may assist individuals who wish to know if they will fit eligibility criteria for particular services and will also provide a list of senior officers who can be approached for further guidance.

Assessment in practice

The evidence from studies of care management of older people is that person-centred assessment is often circumscribed by agency requirements such as the use of checklists, time rationing and inappropriate information technology (IT) systems (Lymbery, 1998; Richards, 2000; Gorman and Postle, 2003). The pressure on throughput in assessments is likely to increase with performance indicators for adult social care that require all assessments to begin within 48 hours of contact and to be completed within four weeks, with 70% of these being completed within two weeks. A new Best Value indicator also requires the provision of services within four weeks following assessment (CSCI, 2006a). Inter-agency working is flagged up within s 47 of the NHS and Community Care Act 1990. Where the assessment discloses a possible housing need or health care need, the relevant primary care trust (PCT) or health authority, or local housing authority shall be invited to assist "to such extent as is reasonable in the circumstances". Section 47(2) of the 1990 Act also requires assessors to identify any disability issues and thus acts as a gateway to the provision of services under s 2 of the Chronically Sick and Disabled Persons Act 1970 (see page 22).

Community care services provision

When the assessment is complete, the local authority will then move on to make the separate 'service provision' decision under s 47(1)(b) of the 1990 Act. Because the provision of such services is rooted in local government, with different local priorities and variable resources, there has been a lack of consistency across the country. This has been exacerbated by the tendency to make less generous provision for older people, particularly in respect of support services for older people to remain in the community. *Fair access to care services* (DH, 2002a) seeks to ameliorate this situation by requiring local authorities not necessarily to provide the same sort of services but to meet the same outcomes for people with similar levels of need. The guidance provides a framework within which local authorities can specify their eligibility criteria, and is based on individuals' needs and associated risks to independence in four eligibility bands: critical, substantial, moderate and low.

- *Critical:* when life or vital social roles are threatened, or significant health problems have developed, or where there is serious abuse or neglect.
- *Substantial:* when choice or control over the immediate environment is substantially limited, for example by an inability to carry out the majority of personal care tasks or domestic routines.
- *Moderate:* when there is, or will be, an inability to carry out several personal care tasks or domestic routines.
- *Low:* when there is, or will be, an inability to carry out one or two personal care tasks or domestic routines.

However, it is up to an individual local authority to decide how high a person's 'eligible needs' have to be before they receive a service. This may mean that services are effectively limited to those in the critical and substantial bands. Once the individual's eligible needs have been established, the local authority must meet those needs (DH, 2002a, para 13). It is not only immediate needs that may be 'eligible' needs; prevention and longer-term needs should also be considered within the criteria. Nor should the local authority impose further eligibility criteria for specific services such as day care, or respite care; there should only be one eligibility decision for all adults seeking social care support, that is, should people be helped or not? Eligibility for help should not depend on age or 'user group' devised for administrative convenience, but should achieve equivalent outcomes, for example sustainability of support systems or control over the immediate environment, for people with similar assessed needs. Eligibility criteria should be published in local 'Better care, higher standards' charters, which are public documents. The success of a prevention agenda depends, however, on resources being allocated to support people at lower levels of need to remain involved with as well as located in their community (DH, 2006a).

Community care services

The sorts of services that may be available are 'community care services' as defined in s 46(3) of the NHS and Community Care Act 1990. These are services such as domiciliary care, day care or residential care, or more broadly, social work support services, provided under the following legislation:

- Part III of the National Assistance Act 1948;
- s 45 of the Health Services and Public Health Act 1968;
- s 21 and Schedule 8 of the NHS Act 1977; and
- s 117 of the Mental Health Act 1983.

Although the Chronically Sick and Disabled Persons Act 1970 is not included in this list, it is referred to indirectly through the reference to Part III of the National Assistance Act 1948, which in s 29 gives local authorities the power to provide services to people with a disability. Because s 46(3) of the NHS and Community Care Act 1990 relies entirely on pre-1990 legislation to provide services, it is arguable that the impact of the 1990 Act has been limited to the duty to assess for pre-existing categories of services. In this sense, the Act can be seen as a case of 'old wine in new bottles', and will not itself support the development of innovative services provision that is responsive to changing user needs.

These particular service provisions are now considered in more detail. Attention should be paid to the distinction between powers and duties, or services the local authority must provide to those who are eligible and services that the local authority may provide if it has the resources to do so.

Residential care

Under s 21 of the National Assistance Act 1948 local authorities have a power to provide residential accommodation "for persons aged 18 and over who by reasons of age, illness or disability, or any other circumstances are in need of care and attention which is not otherwise available to them". Accommodation thus provided is often referred to as 'Part III accommodation'. The Secretary of State's approvals and directions under s 21 of the National Assistance Act 1948 are contained in LAC (93)10 (DH, 1993a), and effectively transform this power into a duty in respect of certain classes of people. The Secretary of State directs local authorities to make arrangements for residential accommodation to persons 'ordinarily resident' in their area and to provide *temporary* accommodation to persons in urgent need. People who suffer from mental disorder receive special mention, with a direction for people ordinarily resident in the area and for those with no settled residence, and an approval in respect of people who, following discharge from hospital, have become resident in the authority's area. A number of beds are usually set aside for what is known as 'short-term care' for simply a week or two weeks to provide respite or a short break, and this may be available on a regular basis.

In addition, the local authority may provide residential care to people of no settled residence, and those who are resident in the area of another authority, with the consent of that authority. Although s 115 of the Immigration and Asylum Act 1999 introduced a new subsection (1A) into s 21 of the National Assistance Act 1948, preventing local authorities from providing residential accommodation to asylum seekers whose need for care and attention had arisen solely because of destitution, there is a continuing responsibility to asylum seekers who are aged and infirm (see *Westminster London Borough Council v NASS* [2002] 1 WLR 2956). In fact, their threshold of need may be lower than that of local residents, as there is no alternative accommodation 'otherwise available' to them, So in *R (on the application of Mari) v Lambeth London Borough Council* [2003] EWCA Civ 836, an asylum seeker with a congenital deformity of the limbs and mental health problems, who could not receive mainstream welfare benefits or council housing, successfully argued that he could have his care needs met only if the local authority provided him with accommodation.

A social work service

Local authorities are directed by the Secretary of State to provide a service for people with disabilities (s 29 of the National Assistance Act 1948) and are approved (by Circular 19/71) to provide visiting and advisory services and social work support to older people under s 45 of the Health Services and Public Health Act 1968. Circular LAC (93)10 (DH, 1993a) directs local authorities to provide social work and related services to help in the diagnosis, assessment and social treatment of mental disorder and to provide social work support to people in their own homes under s 21 of the NHS Act 1977. The provision of social work services (albeit undefined) is thus derived from a statutory basis.

Home help and home care

The provision of home care services is also governed by different pieces of legislation for different user groups, and uses different terminology in different contexts. The statutory provision with the widest scope is para 3(1) of Schedule 8 to the NHS Act 1977. This states:

> It is the duty of every local authority social services authority to provide on such a scale as is adequate for the needs of the area, or to arrange for the provision on such a scale as is adequate, of home-help for households where such help is required owing to the presence of a person who is suffering from illness, lying-in, an expectant mother, aged, handicapped as a result of having suffered from illness or by congenital deformity, and every such authority has power to provide or arrange for the provision of laundry facilities for households for which home help is being, or can be, provided under this sub-paragraph.

This duty is wide enough to cover the provision of services to children as well as to adults, and to the whole household, not just the person who is ill. However, it is framed in terms of a 'target' duty, not one that is owed to any particular individual. To find an enforceable duty to provide 'practical assistance in the home' to a disabled person, one must look to s 2 of the Chronically Sick and Disabled Persons Act 1970. Older people who are disabled are likely to be provided with home care services under the Chronically Sick and Disabled Persons Act 1970. This is advantageous as the specific provision in s 45 of the Health Services and Public Health Act 1968 to provide practical assistance in the home to older people, including adaptations, is a mere power. Although the issue has not been tested, it is arguable, in the case of domiciliary services, that what the law requires in terms of 'practical assistance in the home' is nearer to a traditional home help and housework service than the current home care service for personal care. Most older people eligible for services will be 'disabled', even though they may not be receiving services from a dedicated 'disability' team.

Day services

In respect of day care provision there is again a power to provide services to older people but a duty to provide services for people with a disability or mental health need, whatever their age. Under s 29 of the National Assistance Act 1948, there is a direction (given in LAC (93)10; see DH, 1993a) to provide 'whether at centres or elsewhere' facilities for social rehabilitation and for occupational, social, cultural and recreational activities for people with disabilities. This provision has given impetus to the growth of day centres and adult training centres, which have more recently diversified into day services provision that makes greater use of ordinary community facilities. There is a similar direction (also given in LAC (93)10) to provide day centres and training centres for people suffering from mental disorder under the NHS Act 1977.

Other services

Where need is established, meals services are a duty of the local authority under s 2 of the Chronically Sick and Disabled Persons Act 1970, but a power under s 45 of the Health Services and Public Health Act 1968. 'Boarding out' services (adult placement schemes) are also a power under s 45. A fuller range of services is available as a duty under s 2 of the Chronically Sick and Disabled Persons Act 1970 (see page 22).

Aftercare services under s 117 of the Mental Health Act 1983

Social services authorities and health authorities are under a joint duty to provide services to people detained under some sections of the Mental Health Act 1983 for treatment. However, case law has shown that the duty is simply to use best endeavours to make available services such as residential care, and community nursing support is not a duty that is owed to individuals (*R (B) v Camden London Borough Council* [2005] EWHC 1366 (Admin)). It is established that local authorities may not charge for any service under s 117. The joint duty has to be brought formally to an end and this is usually effective through a review called as part of the Care Programme Approach (CPA) (for further information on this see page 74). It is unlikely that people with deteriorating long-term conditions such as dementia will be discharged from s 117 aftercare. It is crucial in the case of such people to specify whether any residential accommodation is provided under s 117 or under s 21 of the National Assistance Act 1948. This is an important instance where the social worker's legal knowledge in challenging an agency's definition of the legal source of its powers may lead to service users not having to pay for a long-term service that should be provided free of charge. (Further detail of the s 117 aftercare duty is given on page 84.)

Disability services

The provision of services for disabled people is governed by s 29 of the National Assistance Act 1948, the Disabled Persons (Services, Consultation and Representation) Act 1986, and the Chronically Sick and Disabled Persons Act 1970. The emphasis of this earlier legislation, which will be described below, was on the assessment of individual need and the provision of services. The Disability Discrimination Act 1995 has, however, introduced an anti-discriminatory element into service provision focusing on equitable access to employment, housing and the provision of goods and services. It is important that a package of care looks beyond statutory services to different ways of meeting need through social inclusion. Particular tools have been developed to inform the assessment process for people with disabilities; foremost among these is person-centred planning emphasising a strength-based approach that links individuals' aspirations to community networks and non-specialist sources of support. In legal terms there are advantages in emphasising entitlements under the disability legislation as this legislation is constructed around duties rather than powers, on an individual level, and on overcoming barriers to accessing services at both an individual and collective level. The separation in social policy and in legislation of older people from disabled people ignores the commonality of many of their concerns (Priestley and Rabiee, 2001).

The legal definition of a disabled person for the purposes of receiving community care services (including direct payments) is contained in s 29 of the National Assistance Act 1948:

> A local authority may, with the approval of the Secretary of State, and to such extent as he may direct in relation to persons ordinarily resident in the area of the local authority, shall make arrangements for promoting the welfare of persons to whom this section applies, that is to say persons aged 18 or over who are blind, deaf and dumb, or who suffer from mental disorder of any description and other persons aged 18 or over who are substantially and

permanently handicapped by illness, injury or congenital deformity or such other disabilities as may be presented by the Minister.

Note that the definition is wide enough to cover those with physical disabilities, learning disabilities or mental health needs. Section 47(2) of the NHS and Community Care Act 1990 links community care assessments to the disability legislation by requiring assessors specifically to carry out an assessment under s 4 of the Disabled Persons (Services, Consultation and Representation) Act 1986, in respect of a person who is disabled 'without being requested to do so'. This means that it is a responsibility of the assessor properly to identify the person as 'disabled'.

Section 1 of the Chronically Sick and Disabled Persons Act 1970 says:

> ... it shall be the duty of every local authority having functions under s 29 of the National Assistance Act 1948 to inform themselves of the number of persons to whom that section applies within their area and of the need for the making by the authority of arrangements under that section for such persons.

This planning duty of the local authority is supported by the requirement to maintain a register of disabled persons. It is not, however, a prerequisite of getting a service to have one's name on the register. Section 9 of the Disabled Persons (Services, Consultation and Representation) Act 1986 requires local authorities to give a disabled person who receives any of its services, details of any services or benefits they or any other organisation provide. This includes information on welfare benefits and imposes a high premium on the knowledge base of social workers working with people with disabilities.

Section 4 of the Disabled Persons (Services, Consultation and Representation) Act 1986 contains a duty to carry out an assessment when requested to do so by a disabled person, their authorised representative or any person who provides a substantial amount of care on a regular basis. When an assessment is being carried out under the NHS and Community Care Act 1990, s 47(2) provides that

> ... if at any time during the assessment of the needs of the person under subsection 1(a) it appears to a local authority that he is a disabled person, the authority shall proceed to

> make such a decision as to the services he requires as is mentioned in s 4 of the Disabled Persons (Services, Consultation and Representation) Act 1986 without his requesting them to do so.

This means that there is an obligation on local authority assessors to identify people as disabled and to inform them of this further assessment to which they are entitled – a rather clumsy way of ensuring that needs are not overlooked.

Service list under s 2 of the Chronically Sick and Disabled Persons Act 1970

The advantage of an assessment under s 4 of the Disabled Persons (Services, Consultation and Representation) Act 1986 is that it is the gateway to the provision of services under s 2 of the Chronically Sick and Disabled Persons Act 1970. Section 2 contains an extensive 'service list' that can act as a checklist for service provision. The duty on the local authority is to 'make arrangements' that they are satisfied are necessary in order to meet the needs of that person (s 2(1)), for the following services:

- the provision of 'practical assistance' in the home (arguably a 'home help' rather than 'home care' service);
- the provision of, or assistance in, obtaining wireless, television, library or similar recreational facilities;
- the provision of recreational facilities outside the home, or assistance in taking advantage of educational facilities;
- the provision of travel facilities or assistance in travelling to services outside the home (thereby creating a duty to provide travel to day services, payments for which will be subject to the limitations of the fairer charging policy guidance (DH, 2001b)) (see page 131);
- the provision of adaptations or any additional facilities 'designed to secure greater safety, comfort or convenience' (occupational therapists will be involved in assessing the need for adaptations, which may be grant aided; see page 23);
- facilitating the taking of holidays;
- the provision of meals, whether at home or elsewhere;
- the provision of assistance in obtaining a telephone, and any special assistance equipment.

So, the older person with a disability is entitled to participate in a complex assessment process, but one that gives access to a wider range of resources. The extent to which local authorities can take resources into account when conducting assessments and determining need under s 2 of the Chronically Sick and Disabled Persons Act 1970 was itself the question before the House of Lords in the *Gloucestershire* case: *R v Gloucestershire County Council ex parte Barry* [1997] AC 584. The case concerned a reduction in the amount of home care and laundry services provided to a number of older disabled people in Gloucestershire following a revision of eligibility criteria. Services were provided under the Chronically Sick and Disabled Persons Act 1970 that, as we have seen, is phrased in terms of a duty. The service users argued that their needs had not changed; only the local authority financial situation had changed. However, the court held that the local authority could set and revise eligibility criteria based on its own assessment of need. It is important that the scope of the judgment is not exaggerated. Resources could not be the only relevant criterion; other factors such as the degree of the person's disability balanced against the benefit they would receive from the service, had to be taken into account. Pressure on resources could not be used as an excuse for taking arbitrary or unreasonable decisions that would expose vulnerable individuals to the risk of harm. Furthermore, individuals were entitled to a reassessment against the new eligibility criteria, which was not properly done by sending out a letter informing them that a change would take place, as Gloucestershire County Council had done.

Following the *Gloucestershire* case, the Department of Health published LASSL (97)13 (DH, 1997b) to explain the effect of the judgment. The guidance makes it clear that there is a continuing obligation to meet the needs of an individual who is eligible for services if they have met the threshold set by the local authority. This means that individuals cannot be refused services simply because demand is likely to exceed supply and the local authority has run out of money at the end of the financial year. This is an important argument when people are placed on a lengthy waiting list after the decision has been taken that they are in need of and eligible for a particular service.

Equipment and adaptations

The Audit Commission, in its (2000a) report *Fully equipped*, found that there was poor coordination in providing community equipment and aids to daily living between health and social care. There were also long delays in being assessed for and receiving equipment that was sometimes unsuitable or inadequate. Equipment from the NHS is generally intended to meet home nursing care needs, such as pressure relief mattresses and commodes, whereas local authorities may provide equipment such as grab rails and raised toilet seats. However, there is no central 'list' that determines which items are provided by which organisation (Easterbrook, 2003). As part of the programme of intermediate care (DH, 2001c) a National Implementation Team was set up to support the development of integrated community equipment services managed and funded by partnership arrangements under the Health Act 1999 (see page 53). The NHS and local authorities are also responsible for the supply of aids and equipment to care homes in their locality as part of community support services.

There have been recent changes to the grants system for housing repairs, improvements and adaptations that will affect many people with disabilities. Before July 2003, local authorities administered separate grants for Renovations, Home Repairs Assistance and Disabled Facilities, following the provisions of the Housing Grants, Construction and Regeneration Act 1996. Renovations Grants could be awarded to remedy inadequate insulation or heating, or to make premises habitable, whereas Home Repairs Assistance was intended to pay for minor but essential repairs or adaptations for those on a low income (Easterbrook, 2003). Local authorities could also provide funding for people to move to more suitable accommodation. Since July 2003, the scheme has become discretionary, and each local authority will decide what, if any, support it will give out of its own funding.

Disabled Facilities Grants remain, however, under Part 1 of the 1996 Act. Detailed guidance is given in Circular 17/96. It is important to note the overlap between social services' and housing department powers. The housing authority is responsible for the administration and payment of the grant. The maximum mandatory grant is £25,000 in England and £30,000 in Wales. Only people who are disabled under the definition in s 29 of the National Assistance Act 1948 are eligible, although they need not be the home owner. Landlords and tenants are also eligible to apply: although council tenants may have the work carried out by the local authority directly, there should be no difference to the service they receive from that received by direct grant applicants. Purposes for which the grant may be given are listed in s 23 as:

- facilitating access;
- making the dwelling safe;

- providing a bedroom, lavatory, bathroom or washbasin for the disabled occupant;
- facilitating the preparation and cooking of food;
- providing or improving a heating system;
- altering access to sources of power, light or heat;
- facilitating access and movement by the disabled person to enable them to care for another person (child or adult) who is normally resident there.

A wide range of adaptations is therefore included, and can be a part of a more general improvement of the property.

The housing authority has then to be satisfied (s 24(3)) that the relevant works are:

- necessary and appropriate to meet the needs of the disabled occupant (for which it must consult the social services authority usually through an occupational therapy assessment); and
- reasonable and practicable, having regard to the age and condition of the building.

Annex 1 to the guidance says that the housing authority should distinguish between what is desirable, based on the legitimate aspirations of the disabled person, and what is actually needed and for which grant support is fully justified. The consideration of what meets the needs of a disabled person can take into account the question of cost, when there are alternative ways of meeting the need (*R v Kirklees Metropolitan Borough Council ex parte Daykin* [1998] 1 CCLR 512). This can include suggesting rehousing. However, once the authority has decided that the works are necessary and appropriate, and reasonable and practicable, it is mandatory to approve the giving of the grant; at this stage resources are not a relevant factor (*R v Birmingham City Council ex parte Taj Mohammed* [1998] 1 CCLR 441).

There are likely, however, to be differences between what the authority will fund and what the disabled person and their family would like. For example, the guidance advises that the building of a new room 'usable for sleeping' should only be grant funded if the adaptation of an existing room is not suitable; in addition, the installation of central heating or adapted cooking facilities should be limited to meeting the needs of the disabled person. Usual practice for a completed application entails a wait for an occupational therapist's assessment on what is necessary and appropriate, and the submission of builders' estimates based on a specification of works. The housing authority then has six months to respond to the application (s 34 of the Housing Grants, Construction and Regeneration Act 1996). Means testing of grants is made only on the resources of the disabled person and their partner (although someone else may own the house) and normally follows Housing Benefit principles to produce an 'affordable loan'. Where grants are not available but there is an assessed need for an adaptation to the property, Clements (2004) explains that the social services authority is under a continuing duty to make arrangements for home adaptations under s 2 of the Chronically Sick and Disabled Persons Act 1970 and that this duty is not discharged by the decision of the housing authority not to make a grant. In such cases, social services can levy charges under s 17 of the Health and Social Services and Social Security Adjudications Act 1983 provided the cost is over £1,000 (SI 2003/196). Help with equipment such as hoists and other installations that do not involve structural work will normally be the responsibility of the social services authority alone.

Importance of the care plan

A care plan is a 'blueprint for action' (DH, 1991a, para 4.2) designed by the social worker and service user, the aim of which is to identify the most appropriate ways of achieving the objectives identified by the assessment of need and incorporate them into an individual care plan. All users in receipt of a community care service should have a care plan (DH, 1991a, para 4.3) even if the assessment of need is a simple one that can be met by a single service. Without a definition of objectives, even for a single service, the functions of monitoring and review become meaningless (McDonald, 2006). Although the guidance does not describe the care plan as a 'contract', there is a clear legal obligation under s 47(1)(b) of the NHS and Community Care Act 1990 to provide services that the older person has been assessed as needing and for which he or she meets the local authority's eligibility criteria. Sedley J in *R v Islington London Borough Council ex parte Rixon* [1998] 1 CCLR 119 explained the importance of the care plan in linking assessment and service provision:

> ... a care plan is the means by which the local authority assembles the relevant information and applies it to the statutory ends, and hence affords good evidence to any enquirer of the due discharge of its statutory duties.

Copies of the care plan should be made available to all users and carers and to service providers with the consent of the service user. Local authorities that are slow to produce care plans following assessment, perhaps because of a shortage of available resources, may be challenged through the complaints procedure, taking advantage of the 28-day time limit contained therein for the local authority to respond to the complaint (Clements, 2004). This is a useful way of chasing up tardy decision making.

The Single Assessment Process guidance (DH, 2002b) states that the detail of the care plan should include the following:

- a summary of identified and eligible needs, the associated risk to independence and the potential for rehabilitation;
- a note whether the service user has agreed the care plan and whether they have consented to information being shared among relevant agencies;
- the objectives of providing help and anticipated outcomes for users, and a summary of how services will impact on needs and risk;
- the strengths that the older person will bring to the situation;
- how risk will be managed, together with a record of the service user's acceptance of risk;
- details of support that carers will provide and the help that they will receive;
- a description of the level and frequency of help that will be provided and agency responsibility for services, including an integrated nursing plan where appropriate;
- any contribution to care costs that users are required to make;
- a contingency plan, monitoring arrangements and a date for review;
- a contact number for the person coordinating the care plan.

There is thus a strong partnership focus to the care plan, and an expectation that services will be outcomes-focused.

Paragraph 52 of the *Fair access to care services* guidance (DH, 2002a) reiterates the local authority's duty:

> Once a council has decided it is necessary to provide services to meet the eligible needs of an individual, it is under a duty to provide those services.

Commissioning services

It is important similarly in the care plan to distinguish needs from services available to meet those needs. Provided the need can properly be met by either of the alternatives, for example, domiciliary care or residential care, the local authority can decide which of the options is the most cost-effective, although it must (a) take the preferences of the service user into account, and (b) not fetter its discretion by imposing a rigid policy that eschews alternatives. What should always be remembered is that care planning is an individualised process, as the *Practitioners' guide* (DH, 1991a, para 4.12) states:

> Care planning should not be seen as matching needs with services 'off the shelf', but as an opportunity to rethink service provision for a particular individual.

The process of commissioning care services needs to balance diversity with economy of scale. It is one of the paradoxes of community care that where local authorities purchase care on behalf of service users, it is the local authority that is the customer or consumer with purchasing power and not the service user himself or herself. Quality assurance works in these circumstances through standardised service specifications and model contracts, so that the frontline worker negotiates only the detail of the individual service to be provided, based on the care plan (Bamford, 2001).

Conversely, the service can be withdrawn if the user unreasonably refuses to comply with the conditions for its use, including, for example, the provision of a safe working environment for home care staff. So in *R v Kensington and Chelsea London Borough Council ex parte Kujtim* [1999] 4 All ER 161, an asylum seeker was properly evicted from hostel accommodation for threatening behaviour. However, once services have been provided they cannot be withdrawn without a proper re-assessment. Although the *Fair access to care services* guidance (DH, 1991a, paras 47-67) states that all care plans should be regularly reviewed, support should only be withdrawn if the local authority is satisfied that the individual's needs will not significantly worsen in the future for a lack of continuing support. As in the *Gloucestershire* case (see above), local authorities may assess service users against newer and more stringent eligibility criteria, but services cannot be reduced to a level at which the person would be placed in 'serious physical risk'. So, in *R v Birmingham City Council, ex parte Killigrew* (2000) 3 CCLR 109, a reduction in services from 12 to 6 hours daily was unacceptable given the continuing needs of the service user. Given the requirement of equitable treatment for older people in the *National service framework for older people* (DH, 2001a), and the generic application of *Fair access to care services* to all adult service user groups, it is important for agencies to ensure that older people are not put at a disadvantage in being offered a more restricted choice or continuity of service compared to younger people.

Targeting resources and unmet needs

It is common nowadays for resource panels, composed of senior managers, to meet to give financial approval for care packages. This may mean that the social worker's proposals for a package of care, or some elements of it, are rejected on grounds of cost. Schwer (2001) points out that it is important in such situations to clarify when and by whom the service provision decision is made. If it is made by the social worker prior to the submission to the panel then it may be too late for the panel to countermand that decision. If it is a decision that is reserved for the panel then the agency's refusal to fund the package based on cost considerations alone may contravene the requirements in the *Gloucestershire* case that the cost is only one of a number of factors to be balanced against benefits and risks. Even if such a balancing act is carried out by the panel, if they do not give proper consideration to the recommendations from one of their own staff who has seen the evidence of need for themselves, there is a risk that their decision making will be seen as irrational. 'Unmet' needs should be recorded in the care plan and used to inform future service planning (Clements, 2004). There appears to be no legal jeopardy in recording unmet needs insofar as the decision on which presenting needs to regard as eligible is that of the local authority (Clements, 2004). However, agreeing unmet need within a care plan may signpost the desirability of preventative services where the person's condition is likely to deteriorate in the near future.

Reviews

Reviews should be undertaken within three months of services being provided or major changes made, and annually thereafter (DH, 1991a, paras 57-64). A review should assess the extent to which the care package as a whole has met the outcomes laid down in the care plan, and should examine the whole spectrum of services, not concentrate on a single resource. All relevant parties should be involved in the review, including the service user, any carer, and purchasers and providers of services. Decisions should be in writing and individuals should be informed of their rights to use the complaints procedure.

The adequacy of reviews of residential provision has been examined by the local government ombudsman (see page 45) in a case involving Essex County Council (05/A/880) (Mitchell, 2006). By making a placement in a care home the local authority could not divest itself of its continuing responsibility to meet an individual's needs. Monitoring of the way in which these needs were being met should therefore be proactive and frequent. By sticking rigidly to its standard review cycle the local authority could be guilty of maladministration by missing out the critical monitoring stage of the care management process (McDonald, 2006).

Direct payments

The law on providing cash instead of care has undergone substantial revision over its brief existence. The Community Care (Direct Payments) Act 1996 first introduced a power to provide direct payments in lieu of community care services in support of a theoretical shift to 'assistance' rather than 'care'. Following pressure from disability groups to enhance user choice and control, some local authorities had already entered into arrangements with voluntary organisations to make money available through 'indirect' or 'third party schemes' (Clements, 2004). In 2000, the Carers and Disabled Children Act extended eligibility to receive direct payments to carers, to parents of disabled children, and to disabled young people aged 16 and 17, and regulations in 2001 enabled people over the age of 65 to receive direct payments (DH, 2001d). The law on direct payments has now been consolidated by the provisions of ss 57 and 58 of the Health and Social Care Act 2001. Regulations under the Act are the Community Care, Services for Carers and Children's Services (Direct Payments) (England) Regulations 2003 (SI 2003/762). They in effect impose a duty, as opposed to a power in the 1996 legislation (now repealed), to make direct payments in respect of 'prescribed persons' who are otherwise eligible for services. The effect of the 2003 regulations in respect of adults can be summarised as follows:

• any person assessed as needing a community care service will be eligible for direct payments to meet their assessed needs. Repayments may be required if money is spent on services other than those the individual has been assessed as needing;

- people who are subject to guardianship or absent from hospital with leave under the Mental Health Act 1983 are not eligible to receive direct payments, nor are those subject to certain criminal justice measures which require them to submit to treatment for their mental condition or drug or alcohol dependency;
- any recipient must "appear to the responsible authority to be capable of managing a direct payment by himself or with such assistance as may be available to him" (reg 2(1)(a));
- reg 6 is more flexible than previous regulations in allowing payments to be secured from close relatives living in the same household, if the authority is satisfied that securing the service from such a person is necessary to meet satisfactorily the prescribed person's need for that service. Close relatives are:

  - spouses and common law partners
  - parents or parents-in-law (or their spouse or partner)
  - sons or daughters (or their spouse or partner)
  - sons-in-law and daughters-in-law (or their spouse or partner)
  - stepson or step-daughter (or their spouse or partner)
  - brother or sister (or their spouse or partner)
  - aunt or uncle (or their spouse or partner)
  - grandparent (or their spouse or partner).

  Meeting cultural or religious needs, or providing services in an isolated area, may be valid arguments for enabling informal carers to be reimbursed through direct payments. There is no restriction on paying close relatives living outside the household;

- payments cannot be used to purchase prolonged periods of residential care; normally more than a four-week period in any 12 months separated by periods of less than four weeks.

The 2003 guidance on direct payments (DH, 2003a) clarifies the meaning of 'willing and able' to receive a direct payment. Although the test is 'capability' in the sense of having the resources and a sufficient focus to manage direct payments, there is considerable discussion within the guidance on the assessment of mental capacity. Paragraph 48 of the guidance says explicitly that:

> Councils should not make blanket assumptions that whole groups of people will or will not be capable of managing direct payments. A council is not under a duty to make a

direct payment if it does not appear to it that the person is capable of managing the payment, or able do so with assistance. However, very many people will be able to do so, in particular, if they have access to help or support.

Support for direct payments

Developing support services independent of the local authority has been acknowledged to be a major factor in the success of direct payments. Such services can help individuals by running a payroll service to deal with wages, tax and national insurance. If an individual has entered into an enduring power of attorney (EPA) (see page 113), then the attorney under the EPA can continue to receive direct payments on their behalf even though their care needs may fluctuate during this time. Direct payment users are legally responsible for the service that they purchase with direct payments; this means that they are not able to access the local authority's complaints procedure if they encounter difficulties with the services that they purchase. If contingency plans fall through, for example if employees are off sick, then the local authority's duty directly to provide services will revive. In any case, the package of care that the individual receives can be split between direct payments and directly provided services, and this may provide a good opportunity to 'try out' the system. Payments may be made on a gross or a net basis, but will be subject to means testing. The amount of the direct payment must be sufficient to purchase the care needed by the recipient of the direct payment; this may be contentious where private agencies' fees are not fully covered by the amount of the direct payment.

The 2003 guidance makes it clear (para 4) that the provision of direct payments is expected to become mainstream: "whenever a person is assessed as needing social care services, a council should check whether there is a duty to make direct payments in respect of that service". Also, "when setting up a direct payment scheme, local councils are encouraged to actively consider how to include people with different kinds of impairments, people from different ethnic backgrounds and people of different ages" (para 9). This may involve developing a flexible commissioning strategy to divert the amount of resources allocated to block contracts (McDonald, 2006).

Research findings

The research evidence is generally very positive. Dawson (2000) recognised the need for 'champions' to get direct payments off the ground, but also saw benefits, in terms of reducing the workload of social services staff by facilitating self-assessment of need. Stainton (2002), in his survey of users of direct payments, found them overwhelmingly positive about direct payments, often speaking of them in emancipatory language. Significantly, users' own experience did not bear out workers' fears of problems in finding staff, risk and health and safety issues. The piece of research about direct payments most related to older people is by Clark et al (2004). It found that older people receiving direct payments reported feeling happier, more motivated and having an improved quality of life. Support services were crucial in enabling older people to use direct payments and needed to be costed in. There were, however, instances of age discrimination in crossing internal local authority administrative boundaries and in assumptions that older people's needs excluded social activities and were focused on 'personal care'. The next stage in policy development beyond direct payments is likely to be the introduction of individual budgets, following pilot schemes in 2005/06. Individual budgets will incorporate income streams from health and housing as well as social care, and will be based on person-centred planning approaches; they are seen as integral to the philosophy of the 2006 White Paper (DH, 2006a) in strengthening the community presence of older people.

Carers' assessments and carers' services

Assessing the needs of carers together with and separately from the needs of those for whom they care has been a theme of community care legislation in the 1990s and beyond. The use of the word 'carer' is not unproblematic; the vast majority of people providing social care are families, friends or neighbours, the majority of whom will continue to care without any 'official' involvement whatsoever. Others will best be seen as supporters of people who are directly in control of their own care needs. In fact the system of community care is built on there being such a group of people able and willing to provide assistance (McDonald, 2006).

The 2001 Census found that in England and Wales there were 5.3 million carers (approximately 10% of the population), caring being defined as:

> ... looking after or giving help or support to family members, friends, neighbours and others because of long term physical or mental ill-health or disability, or problems related to old age.

The amount and type of assistance given varies widely, and to some extent the legislative framework reflects this (Stalker, 2003).

Carers' assessments

The policy guidance on the NHS and Community Care Act 1990 *Community care in the next decade and beyond* (DH, 1990) included a wide definition of carers as 'families, friends and neighbours' who support vulnerable people, and whose preferences should be taken into account in any community care assessment of the person for whom they care. The guidance stated (para 3.28) that "their willingness to continue caring should not be assumed", and this has now been a theme repeated in later legislation and guidance. In 1996 the Carers (Recognition and Services) Act 1995 introduced a statutory right of assessment for a narrower group of people – those who provide or intend to provide a substantial amount of care on a regular basis. Although 'substantial and regular' were not defined in the Act, it is likely that this group would include the 21% of carers who were identified by the 2001 Census as providing 50 or more hours of care per week. The duty to assess is dependent on a request being made, and is limited to informal carers, thus excluding anyone who provides care under a contract of employment or other contract. So-called 'young carers' (Aldridge and Becker, 1993) are also entitled to assessment under this legislation. CI (95)12 (DH, 1995a) defines a young carer as "a child or young person carrying out significant caring tasks and assuming a level of responsibility for another person which would usually be taken by an adult".

The duty under the 1995 Act is to assess the carer's ability to provide and to continue to provide care, and the assessment will be 'taken into account' when deciding on the provision of services for the person for whom they care. It was not until the coming into force of the Carers and Disabled Children Act 2000 that carers were given a free-standing assessment and an opportunity to have services provided directly to them distinct from the community care services provided to the person for whom they are caring. The Carers and Disabled Children Act 2000 is limited to carers aged 16 and over who provide a 'substantial amount of care' (the same terminology) to another individual aged 18 or over. However, there is no requirement under the 2000 Act that the person cared for has agreed to an assessment, thus giving carers access to services in their own right even if the person for whom they are caring is refusing services. The impact of the caring role is then the focus of the assessment, and relates to the question of whether or not the care given is regular and substantial. Procedural issues are set out in the *Practitioners' guide to carers assessment under the Carers and Disabled Children Act 2000* (DH, 2000a) and they include:

• telling carers of their right to request an assessment;
• assessing 'regular and substantial' in the context of the length of time spent caring, age of the carer, demands of other roles as parent or employee, for example;
• the sustainability of the caring role;
• telling carers they can have a friend or advocate present, involving another worker if appropriate;
• respecting confidentiality and separate recording of interviews where conflicts of interest arise; and
• giving opportunities for review.

Separate guidance on *Developing services for carers and families of people with mental illness* (DH, 2002c) explains the ramifications of Standard 6 of the NSF for mental health, which gives carers of people with a mental illness the right to an annual assessment of their caring needs, set out in a care plan. This guidance also refers to carers as 'co-experts', clarifying their status in relation to statutory service providers. Stalker (2003) considers that the role of informal carer has become professionalised, and recent legislation and directions support this view. So, the Carers (Equal Opportunities) Act 2004 requires social services assessors to inform carers of their right to request an assessment and also requires the assessor to take into account the carer's wish to undertake employment or pursue education. Guidance attached to the community care assessment directions 2004 (DH, 2004b) requires a written note to be made if conflicts of interest or confidentiality mean that carers cannot be consulted. Discharge from hospital may also be properly delayed pending a carer's assessment under the Community Care (Delayed Discharges) Act 2003.

Carers' rights

Research shows that the biggest gap is in the provision of information to carers about assessments; Arksey et al (2000) found that knowledge of the legislation was limited; around half of all carers interviewed had not been formally assessed and carers were not routinely provided with a written record of outcomes. With many carers still in employment, 'family-friendly' policies in the workplace may be vital to maintaining this dual role. Section 8 of the Employment Relations Act 1999 has given employees the right to a reasonable amount of time off as unpaid leave to provide assistance to 'dependants' or to deal with unexpected disruptions to their care. Phillips et al (2002) investigated the experiences of carers of older people in the light of such policies. They found that although one in 10 employees were involved in caring for parents or parents-in-law, there was a lack of openness about these caring responsibilities compared to childcare responsibilities. This led to very few employees taking advantage of policies that identified them as 'in need' or 'not coping'. It appears then that there is a need for sensitive publicity to support carers in taking up their right to support when engaged in supporting older relatives or other dependants. If this does not happen, it is likely that services will be offered only in crisis when people who would have liked to have continued caring are no longer able to do so.

Remuneration for carers outside of the benefits system may also be an issue. Whether or not a financial contribution to a family member could be set off against a charge for community care services raised an important principle in *R (Stephenson) v Stockton-on-Tees Borough Council* [2005] WLR (D) 102. Mrs Stephenson wished to pay her daughter for care provided, but the local authority policy was not to set such a payment against assessed charges for home care services unless 'cultural issues' could successfully be argued. It was assumed that family members would give their time without payment. The local authority in that case was told to reconsider its decision taking into account the existence of 'exceptional circumstances' other than cultural issues which the family itself had agreed was the best way of managing Mrs Stephenson's care.

Carers' services

It is of course possible for carers also to be service users of community care services in their own right. A model of mutual support may best represent the type of caring situation that many older people are involved in, based on reciprocity and mutual rewards. Section 2 of the Carers and Disabled Children Act 2000, however, defines 'carers' services' for the purpose of that Act differently from community care services. Carers' services are:

... any services which –

(a) the local authority sees fit to provide; and
(b) will in the local authority's view help the carer care for the person cared for,

and may take the form of physical help or other forms of support.

This may be contrasted with the very tight definition of community care services under s 46(3) of the NHS and Community Care Act 1990. Carers' services may include, for example, help with gardening or the provision of leisure facilities or a mobile phone. Local authorities have wide scope in the use of Carers' Grants to provide services although it should be noted that the provision of carers' services is a power not a duty, so will be constrained by budgets. Some services, for example, night sitting or domiciliary care, may be capable of being seen as either services for carers or services for the person for whom they care. Section 2(3) of the Carers and Disabled Children Act 2000 enables a carer's service to be provided directly to the person being cared for with their consent. The autonomy of the cared-for person is preserved by not allowing such a service to be anything of an intimate nature, except in an emergency. It is easy to imagine a scenario nevertheless where a night sitter, for example, is provided for a reluctant or mentally incapacitated older person, and the night sitter is involved in washing or taking to the toilet the older person for whom they are caring without consent having been explicitly obtained.

Abuse of older people

When carers are under stress, or unsupported, or an older person is vulnerable to harm or exploitation, the potential for abuse may exist. In examining the issue of abuse, we must fall back on general legal principles and remedies often developed in other contexts. Some parallels exist of course with child abuse but it cannot be assumed that similar rights and duties exist, or that similar remedies will be appropriate. The definition of actions or the consequences as abusive is a matter of social construction: is it abusive to lock a person with dementia in their room to prevent them from walking out into a busy road? Is it abusive for a carer under stress to threaten to put the person for whom they care 'in a home'? Is it abusive for a family to use a mobility allowance to purchase a car for their own use? The boundary between abuse and less than optimum care may be difficult to draw, particularly in situations where there is no intention to cause harm, or no criminal act has been committed. The language used to describe the phenomenon itself reflects dilemmas and ambiguities in relation to culpability and vulnerability. The phenomenon of abuse has been described as 'miscare', when the emphasis has been on carer stress, and as 'any action which is an abuse of a person's human rights' when the emphasis has been on the victim. Similarly, there has been a movement away from medico-legal definitions of abuse, to socio-legal definitions of the duty to protect, and, latterly, safeguard (ADSS, 2005).

Policy developments

Although victims of abuse are found across the whole age spectrum, there is evidence that they are disproportionately in the older age groups (McCreadie, 1996). The charity Action on Elder Abuse has become prominent in the field; it publishes a number of useful leaflets and a 24-hour helpline. The Law Commission (1995), in the context of reviewing the law on mental incapacity, looked at the possibility of a public law duty to investigate and respond to abuse but no specific legal duty to investigate has as yet been created to parallel the duty to investigate in s 47 of the Children Act 1989.

No secrets

The publication of policy guidance *No secrets* in 2000 (DH, 2000b) has marked a formulation of adult protection issues not only for older people but also for all vulnerable adults. Any person in need of community care services may be considered to be a vulnerable adult under the guidance if they are unable to protect themselves from harm or exploitation. The guidance defines abuse in very wide terms as interference with a person's personal and human rights. It also adds discriminatory abuse to categories of physical, sexual, psychological and financial abuse and neglect. Although social services authorities are the lead agency under *No secrets*, cases in which there is an initial allegation of criminal activity are to be referred to the police for investigation. Procedures for the investigation of alleged abuse parallel child protection processes with scope for inter-professional strategy meetings and case conferences and the drawing up of protection plans. Research by Preston-Shoot and Wigley (2002) found that there was a continuing need for raising awareness of the prevalence of abuse particularly in non-specialist agencies such as housing. Recent guidance from the Association of Directors of Social Services also emphasises inter-agency responsibilities and the importance of 'safeguarding' vulnerable adults by preventative action as well as by the strengthening of investigative procedures (ADSS, 2005).

Legal responses

Adults with mental capacity (see page 66) may make reasoned decisions to accept abusive situations rather than risk losing their home and family. This makes the choice of intervention strategies particularly difficult. Elder abuse in some contexts may be the outcome (continuation or role reversal) of domestic violence which has existed for some years and only becomes visible when one of a couple becomes frailer or more visible to outside agencies. Just as elder abuse covers a wide range of different situations and circumstances, so the appropriateness of the legal response will vary. Police experience in domestic violence units has in some areas been extended to the abuse of vulnerable adults. The protection of domestic violence legislation has been extended beyond spouses living in the matrimonial home by Part IV of the Family Law Act 1996. That Act enables non-molestation orders and occupation orders to be obtained against 'associated persons', which includes relatives and those living in the same household, for example, adult children. The initiative, however, rests with the applicant, who may be in need of support. Those who are incapacitated from taking action on their own behalf may act through the Official Solicitor. Injunctions may also be available in other civil proceedings, for example, in an action for trespass or assault. The Domestic Violence, Crime and Victims Act 2004 brings together civil and criminal remedies by making breach of a non-molestation order a criminal offence. Also, in s 6 the Act introduces a specific new offence of causing or allowing the death of a vulnerable child or adult whether by direct action or by a failure to protect. Anti-Social Behaviour Orders, introduced by the Crime and Disorder Act 1998, may be used to deter sub-criminal behaviour perceived as threatening by older people; such orders may be applied for by the police or by the local authority or by housing authorities. The Protection from Harassment Act 1997, which can be both punitive and protective, enables restraining orders to be made (s 5) for the protection of older people who are being harassed on a continuing basis. One difficulty may lie in obtaining sufficient reliable evidence from witnesses who may be mentally or physically infirm, and who are reluctant to press charges. Implementation of Part II of the Youth Justice and Criminal Evidence Act 1999 has extended to vulnerable adults measures designed to protect child witnesses. These include the opportunity to video record evidence, and the use of protective screens in court.

The use of enduring powers of attorney or appointment of a receiver to deal with the financial affairs of older people may be a preventative measure worth taking (see Chapter Four, this volume, for details). Contracts entered into by people who are incapacitated will be voidable at the behest of the mentally incapacitated person, unless they are for necessaries such as food and shelter. It is also possible to set aside contracts for 'mistake' or to unravel 'unconscionable bargains', such as the sale of valuables for far below their obvious market value. (see McDonald and Taylor, 1995). It is worth taking legal advice in these circumstances.

Cases of neglect, however, pose particular difficulties. In order to found a remedy in a case of neglect, it is first of all necessary to find a person who owes a duty to the elderly victim of that neglect. While parents owe a duty to their infant children, children and other family members do not conversely owe a legal duty to elderly parents. It is otherwise if a duty is voluntarily assumed; civil liability will exist in the law of tort for the negligent breach of that duty, and if there is gross neglect then there may well be criminal liability as well. Section 44 of the Mental Capacity Act 2005 (due to be implemented from April 2007) makes it a criminal offence to ill-treat or neglect a person for whom one acts as a lasting power of attorney (see page 67) or any person who is incapacitated who is under one's care. The standard of care that the courts have demanded has in fact been quite high and the greater the risks, the higher the standard of care. Constant supervision may thus be required, particularly in an institutional context, in the case of people such as the elderly mentally infirm, who pose particular risks. If a duty of care is found to exist, then it is no defence for the defendant to say that they would have found it difficult because of their own limitations properly to fulfil that duty; the test is an objective one – what would a reasonable person in the circumstances have done?

Although there may be a range of established legal options available using criminal or civil law, the context in which any assessment should take place is that of s 47 of the NHS and Community Care Act 1990. Adult protection should be seen therefore in terms of support to vulnerable individuals, rather than as a reaction to abuse; this parallels developments in childcare from protection to safeguarding of children's rights and family support.

Compulsory removal from home

Outside of the Mental Health Act 1983, compulsory removal from home for people not suffering from mental disorders is governed by the principles of s 47 of the National Assistance Act 1948. This archaic (and ageist) piece of legislation enables the 'proper officer' (community physician or public health specialist) to apply to a magistrates' court for removal to hospital, residential care, or any other suitable place. This therefore is a judicial process unlike the largely administrative process of admission under the Mental Health Act. But there is no requirement that the person should be brought before the court, or be legally represented. The grounds for removal are that the person is:

> Suffering from grave, chronic disease or being aged, infirm or physically incapacitated is living in insanitary conditions, and is unable to devote to himself and is not receiving from other persons proper care and attention. (s 47(1))

The community physician has to provide a certificate that it is either in the interests of the person concerned, or for the prevention of injury to the health of, or serious nuisance to, other persons that the elderly person is removed. So, for example, a person whose house is full of hoarded garbage, or infested with vermin may be threatened with removal for the protection of neighbours. Alternatively, it would be possible to construe s 47 as applicable in cases of abuse where proper care is not being provided, There is an emergency procedure under s 1 of the National Assistance (Amendment) Act 1951 for removal in an emergency without giving the seven days' notice required under the 1947 Act. In this case, two medical opinions are needed and the initial period of removal is for three weeks, not for three months as it is under the 1947 Act. The decision to remove is usually preceded by a case conference, and although there are only about 200 cases of removal each year, the provision may be invoked as a means of bringing agencies together to look at a complex, deteriorating situation. Powers to enter and fumigate property under the Environmental Protection Act 1990 may be invoked at the same time. Importantly, there should be a care plan for an eventual return home, lest continuing use of residential care leads to a permanent admission by default. If there is evidence of a mental disorder, the procedurally more robust Mental Health Act should be considered, and BASW (British Association of Social Workers) advises social workers to become involved in s 47 proceedings only if removal would positively contribute to the individual's well-being, both physical and mental. The lack of procedural safeguards and the disproportionate impact of removal from home make s 47 vulnerable to challenge under the Human Rights Act 1998. Although reform of the law was considered by the Law Commission in its *Mental incapacity report* (1995), there are no current proposals to replace s 47. The European Court of Human Rights has also upheld similar legislation in Switzerland based on vagrancy laws, seeing such legislation as ultimately necessary for the protection (and control) of vulnerable adults (*HM v Switzerland* (2002) Application 39187/98, European Court of Human Rights).

Resolving disputes

Some of the most difficult cases concern family conflict over the care of an older person. Here the issue may not be intentional abuse, but a lack of satisfactory care, or simply a dispute about the best interests of the vulnerable adult. For example, family members or professionals may disagree about whether a vulnerable person should remain at home, or should be admitted to residential care. Although the Children Act 1989 provides a range of orders applicable to children, including Emergency Protection Orders, Care Orders and 'Section 8' Orders dealing with residence or contact or specific issues, there has been no parallel legislation for the protection of vulnerable adults who are unable to make decisions for themselves. To cover this gap in the law, the High Court has developed its power to grant declaratory relief into the field of adult protection to make decisions about contact and residence. So, in *Re S (Hospital Patient: Court's Jurisdiction)* [1996] Fam 1, a declaration was granted that it was in the best interests of an elderly man incapacitated by a stroke to remain in hospital in England; the court also granted an injunction to prevent his family, who lived in Norway, from removing him from the jurisdiction. In *Re F (Adult: Court's Jurisdiction)* [2000] 3 WLR 1740, the Court of Appeal granted a declaration that it was in the best interests of a young woman with learning disabilities to remain in their care rather than return to her family; the court also placed restrictions on contact with her mother. The use of this power on a case-by-case basis is clearly unsatisfactory, but remains a possible remedy until the implementation of the Mental Capacity Act 2005 (see page 66) provides a statutory basis for decision making.

Challenging decisions

When statutory services are provided or decisions made, there are a number of ways in which decisions can be challenged, depending on the outcome that is wanted. This may be simply an apology, a change in service, compensation or a change in policy or procedure. Remedies may be pursued internally within the agency, or by reference to outside agencies or the courts. Advocacy or advisory services may be available to assist people in pursuing complaints.

Local authority complaints procedures

Local authorities are required to have complaints procedures to deal both with children's services and with community care services. In respect of community care services, s 50 of the NHS and Community Care Act 1990 amends s 7 of the Local Authority Social Services Act 1970 to enable the Secretary of State to direct local authorities to set up procedures for considering representations, including complaints. The Complaints Procedure Directions 1990 and Department of Health guidance *The right to complain* (1991b) established the procedure to be followed.

Complaints should be brought within 12 months and must be made by or on behalf of a 'qualifying individual'. A person is a qualifying individual if:

> ... a local authority has a power or a duty to provide, or to secure the provision of, a social service for him or her; and his or her need for such a service has (by whatever means) come to the attention of the local authority. (DH, 2006e, para 2.4.1)

There is also a discretion to deal with complaints or representations outside these categories. Complaints procedures should be kept separate from grievance procedures and disciplinary procedures that concern internal staffing matters.

Stages within a local authority complaints procedure

The procedures themselves are in three stages: an informal stage, a formal stage and a review panel stage. Under the original procedures, a formal written complaint becomes a 'registered' complaint to which the authority should respond within 28 days. Complaints concerning independent providers that cannot be resolved within the provider's own internal complaints procedure are to be referred to the local authority as registered complaints. If the complainant informs the authority within 28 days of the notification of the outcome of the formal stage, that he or she is still dissatisfied and requests the complaint to be referred to a panel for review, the local authority is required to convene a panel to meet within 28 days of the request. The panel will be chaired by a person who is independent of the local authority. Complainants are entitled to make written formal submissions and are also entitled to an oral hearing. They may be accompanied by a supporter or advocate, although legal representation is not normally allowed. Although the panel hearing is 'informal', it must conform to the principles of natural justice and to the requirements of a 'fair hearing' within Article 6 of the European Convention on Human Rights. Access to files may need to be requested in advance, as the time limit for the local authority to respond to such a request is a lengthy 40 days.

The panel operates by way of rehearing the complaint, and is essentially a fact-finding body. It does not have the expertise to examine complex legal issues, which may then go straight to judicial review. However, its recommendations may extend to changing local authority policy and it can ask the local authority to report back on subsequent changes made. Panels can also recommend that successful claimants should receive modest compensation for distress (usually a maximum of £2,000 per year) and for time and trouble in bringing the complaint (usually in the range of £25 to £250). Although the panel's recommendation is not binding, it cannot be overruled 'without substantial reason' (*R v Avon CC, ex parte M* [1994] 2 FLR 1006). The operation of local authority complaints procedures comes within the jurisdiction of the local government ombudsman (see below) whose reports show concern about undue delay, unfairness and failure in sensitive cases to use independent advocates to assist complainants.

The role of the Commission for Social Care Inspection

Following a Department of Health consultation *Listening to people* (DH, 2000c), the Commission for Social Care Inspection (CSCI) assumes responsibility for the review of complaints about local authority social services departments under the Health and Social Care (Community Health and Standards) Act 2003. The intention is to harmonise procedures for dealing with complaints relating to children with those relating to adults. A complaints manager within the local authority will oversee a two-stage internal process of local resolution (for which a 10-day time limit is proposed) and formal investigation (involving an investigating officer from the local authority and with a time limit of 25 days). Following this, a senior service manager must respond to the complainant, in a process to be known as 'the adjudication' to say what action the authority is intending to take to address the outcome of the investigation. A complainant who remains dissatisfied may request an independent review within two months before a complaints panel of three independent people convened by CSCI. CSCI can also investigate where the substance of the complaint and the local process for investigating complaints gives rise to concern. It can also refer the complaint back to local resolution or onwards to the ombudsman.

The consultation proposes that there should be a presumption in favour of deferring changes to any care plan while the complaints procedure is in operation. It also proposes that duties of cooperation or lead authority status should be used to resolve disputes concerning complex cases where both health and social care are involved. When the quality of care homes provision is the issue, complaints to CSCI may also be made under the Care Standards Act 2000 about breaches of regulations or minimum standards, and to the local authority about the placement's failure to provide an adequate standard of care, with coordination between the two processes to give a combined response. Regulations and guidance have now been issued (DH, 2006e) to give effect to the outcomes of the consulation.

Ombudsmen

The idea of 'ombudsmen' to investigate complaints of maladministration in public services comes from Scandinavia and was first introduced into England and Wales in 1967. The system now covers both central and local government as well as the NHS, and it has also extended into the commercial field (McDonald, 1997). The function of the ombudsman is to uphold principles of good administration, fairness and competence, not to question the merits of a decision – for that the complaints procedure should be used. If the legality of a decision is in question, then judicial review is the appropriate remedy. Complaints must be made within 12 months, but where the complainant is unable to apply in person, a representative may do so on their behalf. The ombudsman acts by an inquisitorial process and has the power to command documents and the appearance of witnesses. Modest amounts of compensation may be ordered to be paid to those who have suffered injustice as a consequence of maladministration. An innovation has been for the ombudsman in some cases to require local authorities to report back to them in three months' time on progress made in reforming systems. The health service ombudsman has made a significant impact on the development of policy, as well as good practice, particularly in the field of continuing care. Case number E22/02-03 'The Pointon Case', involving the former Cambridgeshire Health Authority and South Cambridgeshire PCT (available at www.ombudsman.org.uk), explained the applicability of continuing NHS care services to people in the community and their link with direct payments (see page 60) thus linking health care and social care issues.

Default powers

In the field of public law, if a local authority fails to carry out any of its statutory duties, s 7D of the Local Authority Social Services Act 1970 enables the Secretary of State to declare the authority to be in default, issue directions to ensure that the duties specified are complied with, and, if necessary, enforce those directions in the High Court. The invocation of the default power may be a prerequisite to a private law remedy, as in *Wyatt v Hillingdon London Borough Council* [1978] 76 LGR 727, where the dispute concerned an alleged breach of the duty under s 2 of the Chronically Sick and Disabled Persons Act 1970 to provide an adequate amount of home care. Most disputes are likely to be about the provision of resources from central government to local government, so in *R v Westminster City Council ex parte P and others* [1998] 1 CCLR 486, a dispute concerning the resettlement of destitute asylum seekers was held not to be an appropriate matter for the courts but for the exercise of the political discretion of the Secretary of State. The administrative equivalent of the use of default powers is provided by the Local Government Act 2000, which enables the Secretary of State to place local authorities under 'special measures' or allow their functions to be taken over by other authorities when performance indicators have not been met.

Monitoring officer

In order to scrutinise policy or decisions for illegality or maladministration, every local authority is required by s 5 of the Local Government and Housing Act 1989 to appoint a monitoring officer. This function is often carried out by the local authority's chief executive or the head of its legal department. Drawing the monitoring officer's attention to the issue in dispute may thus be a useful first step in trying to get policy changed or a decision reversed before further formal action to challenge its legality is taken.

Legal actions

Historically, recipients of community care services have not been prominent in taking legal action and the law in this area has not been well developed. However, there is certainly scope for challenging the propriety of assessments, the rationing of resources and the quality of services. Because community care legislation is so minimalist, usually providing only a framework for decision making, differences of interpretation and policy will certainly arise, leading to challenges. Also, the implementation of the Human Rights Act 1998 provides another avenue of challenge against the actions of public authorities that supports claims for equality of opportunity and treatment. The desire not to set an unwelcome legal precedent may be a spur to compromise on the part of the authority whose decision is challenged. This is certainly an area in which legal advice will be needed, but for further discussion on the scope and range of remedies, see McDonald (1997).

Actions for breach of statutory duty

As the duties of local authorities are the creation of statute, it may be thought that breaches of those duties would be actionable by potential service users most affected by them. This is not in fact the case. An action for breach of statutory duty will exist only if the statute can be construed as intending to give rise to an individual right of action, and most duties to make services available in their area are seen as 'target' duties, where local authorities have a discretion concerning the quantity and range of services that they provide. Although s 2 of the Chronically Sick and Disabled Persons Act 1970 was construed in the *Gloucestershire* case (see page 23) as giving a personal right of action to anyone whose need for services was not met, the duty on the health authority to provide support from a psychiatrist under s 117 of the Mental Health Act 1983 has been construed as a duty only 'to use its best endeavours'. This is so, even if the support has been specified by a mental health review tribunal (*R (H) v Secretary of State for the Home Department and others* [2003] 3 WLR 1278).

Actions in negligence

Actions in negligence seeking compensation by way of damages may be available against individuals, or against corporate bodies if there can be shown to be a breach of a duty of care. Under the Mental Health Act 1983, liability is personal to the approved social worker making the application for admission (see page 77), but he or she is protected from criminal or civil liability by s 139 of the Act unless there is proof of bad faith or lack of reasonable care, and civil proceedings in such cases require leave of the High Court. In other cases where failure to meet a reasonable standard of care is alleged, employers will be vicariously liable for the actions of their staff performed in the course of their employment. It was accepted in *Carty v Croydon London Borough Council* [2005] EWCA Civ 19 that such a duty of care extended to those such as education officers who did not have professional qualifications.

The limits of liability in cases involving complex policy decisions have been contested. In *Barrett v Enfield London Borough Council* [2001] 2 AC 550, the House of Lords accepted that there could be liability where social workers had failed to gather proper information or follow through review decisions in relation to children in their care. This was 'negligence in an operational manner' which could be distinguished from the courts' reluctance (at that time) to find that the local authority was liable for negligence in respect of policy decisions, such as the decision to take child protection proceedings. Substantial inroads have more recently been made to this principle. In *W and others v Essex County Council and another* [2000] 2 All ER 237, the local authority was held liable for failing fully to disclose the background of a child whom it had placed with foster carers in circumstances where the child went on to abuse the foster carers' own children. The European

Court of Human Rights in *Z and others v UK* (2002) 34 EHRR 3 has also found that there was a breach of Article 3 as well as Article 13 in the failure to protect vulnerable children by the proper use of child protection procedures as well as in the failure to provide a mechanism by which individuals could receive a remedy in damages for this breach. This was a direct challenge to the decision of the House of Lords, in *X (Minors) v Bedfordshire County Council* [1995] 3 All ER 353, that a local authority was immune from a claim in negligence on the basis that 'general policy decisions' are not justiciable. The way is open therefore in future cases to argue not only that the European Convention on Human Rights requires remedies in negligence to be developed to cover policy as well as operational issues, but also that Article 3 requires the development of effective forms of protection against 'cruel, inhuman and degrading treatment' suffered by vulnerable adults as well as children.

Judicial review

Judicial review provides a remedy in public law, rather than private law. Applications for review are brought in the Administrative Court Office of the Queen's Bench Division of the High Court. The application is for the review of decisions made, not an appeal. Only bodies that perform public functions are subject to judicial review, but that includes local authorities, health care bodies, universities and professional regulatory bodies. The applicant has to have a sufficient interest in the matter in question to show 'standing', but group actions have been successfully brought by bodies such as RADAR and Help the Aged. The grounds for judicial review are: illegality (acting ultra vires, or beyond one's powers); procedural impropriety (or not following 'due process' in proceedings); and irrationality (making a decision that no reasonable body could make). Judicial review proceedings have established some basic principles of decision making:

- that all relevant matters should be taken into account (for example, medical evidence provided to support the applicant's case), but irrelevant matters should be disregarded (such as the ability to purchase a service privately);
- that prior consultation should take place with people who will be affected by the decision (such as the closure of a residential home);
- that decision makers should be objective and not have a personal interest in the outcome of the decision, although 'administrative'

decision making is acceptable by, for example, allocation panels for community care services;
- that 'legitimate expectations' should be met in terms of the process to be used for making decisions (for example, published criteria for assessments or eligibility for services) and appropriate guidance followed;
- that generally reasons should be given for decisions made.

Normally, leave is required to bring judicial review proceedings and other remedies must have been exhausted. Proceedings usually need to be brought within three months of the cause of action arising, although when the complaint is one of a continuing breach of a statutory duty, time limits are unimportant. Negotiations may have to take place with the body whose decision is being challenged, either to adjourn an application for judicial review while other remedies are being pursued, or to obtain a guarantee that an out-of-time argument will not be taken. An application for judicial review can be used as a campaigning tool, as well as a strictly legal remedy (McDonald, 1997).

The orders that can be made in judicial review proceedings are discretionary. They are mandatory orders (to compel a public authority to carry out its duty); quashing orders (to require the authority to make a new decision); and prohibitory orders (to prevent a particular course of action). The court may also make a declaration that states the law (for example, on the legality of medical treatment), or issue a mandatory injunction to ensure provision is continued.

European dimension

The coming into force of the Human Rights Act 1998 in October 2000 has enabled a new cause of action to be brought against public authorities under s 7 for breaches of Convention rights. An alleged breach of Convention rights can also be used as a defence when legal actions are brought against individuals. The British Institute of Human Rights (2002) has argued that the success of the Human Rights Act for older people will be dependent on judgments being made that there are also active positive duties to promote the welfare of older people not simply duties to respond to threats of abuse. In the context of community care this will necessitate a greater willingness to scrutinise resource provision decisions and challenge discriminatory action, than has been apparent before.

Case study 1: Carer's assessment

Jane Allen is 55 years old and works part time in a supermarket. When her father died suddenly two years ago she moved in with her 88-year-old mother, Ruth, who has Alzheimer's Disease. Jane helps Ruth with washing and dressing and does all the cooking and cleaning. She is often woken at night by Ruth who is restless and agitated when she is left alone. Jane would like to retain her job, but on several occasions has been called home by neighbours who have telephoned to say that Ruth is wandering in the street. Jane's boss tells her that her job is at risk if she takes any more time off work. Jane is adamant that she still wants to look after Ruth at home, but wonders how much longer she can manage.

What sort of services might be available to Ruth in these circumstances and what are Jane's rights as a carer?

To what extent does the legal framework support good social work practice in this sort of situation?

Further reading

McDonald, A. (2006) *Understanding community care: A guide for social workers* (2nd edn), Basingstoke: Palgrave.
Looks at the history and development of community care for all user groups, not just older people. Explains the process of care management from a social work and research perspective but emphasises throughout the legal framework within which community care has been developed.

Clements, L. (2004) *Community care and the law* (3rd edn), London: Legal Action Group.
A comprehensive account of community care law that makes specific reference to the law relating to older people. This is an excellent reference work and contains in appendices extracts from the key pieces of legislation and guidance.

Easterbrook, L. (2003) *Moving on from community care: The treatment, care and support of older people in England*, London: Age Concern.
Surveys the development of community, residential and health care services for older people, with an emphasis on the translation into practice of law and policy. Provides a good foundation for challenging decision making in individual cases, by emphasising good practice.

TWO

Health care needs

Many service users have specific health care needs as well as social care needs, and inter-agency and inter-professional working is fundamental to the effective delivery of a cohesive package of care. The 'internal market' that was a feature of health care in the 1990s has more recently been replaced by that of partnership both between health care bodies and between the NHS and social care, and the introduction of private finance initiatives (PFIs) has brought private health care directly into the NHS. Part III of the Health and Social Care Act 2001, although little used, has enabled the creation of care trusts as separate legal entities to combine responsibility for the discharge of health and social care functions. The more commonly used s 31 of the Health Act 1999 introduced new opportunities to pool budgets or transfer resources by the creation of 'Health Act flexibilities'. Such flexibilities may be used for the development of whole services or individual packages of care. There are three ways in which this can be done: pooled funded arrangements (for example, where community nurses may commission social care services such as home care and day care); lead commissioning (such as, for example, that all mental health services are commissioned by a single health care body); and integrated provision (where both health and local authority services are provided by a single provider under one management). Generally, s 27 of the Health Act 1999 says that "In exercising their respective functions NHS bodies (on the one hand) and local authorities (on the other) shall co-operate with one another in order to secure and advance the health and welfare of the people of England and Wales".

The desire for uniformity in service provision to meet identified health care priorities was exemplified in the development of national service frameworks (NSFs). Principles of the NSFs for mental health, for older people and for long-term care may all be applicable to older people, and services will be developed according to these standards. Also influential for health care planning is the White Paper on public health (DH, 2004a). The focus is on prevention and encouraging healthier lifestyles. Following the Evercare model in the US, modern matrons carrying out functions similar to those of care managers will identify and encourage expert patients to monitor their own health and use of medication. The target group is people with complex needs – three or more long-term conditions – a group that will include many older people. Private responsibility for health care decisions has become embodied in this way in policy initiatives that focus resources predominantly in the community rather than in institutional provision.

Legal basis of NHS care

Despite these 'modernising changes', the basic premise of the NHS remains, that it should be a universal service funded out of general taxation and free (generally) at the point of delivery. There is potential for conflict therefore in practice between these principles and the selective, means-tested provision of social care services. The governing statute for NHS care remains the National Health Service Act 1977, which lays down basic powers and duties for the provision of health care both in hospitals and in the community. Section 1(1) of the Act provides:

> It is the Secretary of State's duty to continue the promotion in England and Wales of a comprehensive health service designed to secure improvement – in the physical and mental health of the people of those countries, and in the provision, diagnosis and treatment of illness, and for that purpose to provide and secure the effective provision of services in accordance with this Act.

The 1977 Act goes on to say how this may be done – by giving the Secretary of State a duty to provide hospital, medical, dental, nursing and ambulance services, and such facilities for the prevention, care and aftercare of illness as he considers "necessary to meet all reasonable requirements" (s 3). This duty, so widely framed, is a target duty and no more; it is not enforceable, the courts have decided, by means of a legal action by individuals. Questions of resource allocation remain in the political sphere. So, in *R v Secretary of State for Social Services, ex parte West Midlands Health Authority and Birmingham Area Health Authority, ex parte Hincks* [1980] 1 BMLR 93, the Court of Appeal refused to interfere with the decision to close a local renal unit on the application of patients who were then faced with a longer journey for their treatment. The courts will, however, intervene if the health care body to which the Secretary of State has delegated decision-making powers fails to consult properly, or develops policies which permit it to disregard clear duties within the National Health Service Act 1977. Both of these issues were discussed in the context of NHS responsibilities for continuing care in the *Coughlan* case (see below). Even guidance from the Secretary of State will be unlawful if it has the effect of diluting a legal duty.

Since April 2004 the Healthcare Commission has carried out performance monitoring in the NHS by means of an annual audit while NICE, the National Institute for Clinical Excellence, advises the NHS on treatment options and prescribing. Local authority scrutiny of NHS functions is undertaken by overview and scrutiny committees comprising elected members. There is thus a complex array of mechanisms for formal scrutiny of NHS functions and resource allocation decisions. At an individual practitioner level, the regulatory powers of professional bodies are overseen by a new Council for the Regulation of Healthcare Professionals, set up in consequence of the Bristol Child Heart Deaths inquiry (Kennedy, 2001) as an end to professional hegemony in the investigation of malpractice.

Responsibility for community health care

Most people receive care solely from primary health care teams organised around general medical practitioner partnerships. The terms of service of GPs as independent practitioners within the NHS have recently changed with the introduction of a new General Medical Services contract, which enables GPs to manage their personal workload according to their interests and patients' needs, while ending the previously obligatory out-of-hours requirement. Everyone living in the UK has the right to register with a GP practice, although there is no right to be treated by a particular GP within the practice. There is a right to see a GP within two working days or another health care professional within one working day (Easterbrook, 2005). The decision to visit at home or to refer to a consultant is that of the GP; there is no right to such a service. The local primary care trust (PCT) is required to provide general practice services to those unable to register with a GP.

Some GP practices may also choose to deliver so-called 'enhanced' services, such as minor surgery, which cross the boundary between secondary and primary care. Primary care is also responsible for the delivery of community health care services to people in care homes, as well as those living in their own accommodation. Since s 49 of the Health and Social Care Act 2001 has prohibited local authorities from providing nursing care by a registered nurse as a community care service (whether in a residential setting or otherwise), the provision of nursing care is the financial responsibility of the PCT. The application of the three bands of the Registered Nursing Care Contribution (RNCC), which assesses the amount of care provided by or under the direction of a registered nurse, and quantifies the NHS contribution to the resident's care, is described in HSC 2001/17 (DH, 2001g).

The distinction drawn between health and social care responsibilities in the *Coughlan* case (see below) was applied in *R (D) v Haringey London Borough Council* [2005] EWHC 2235 (Admin), to a dispute between the local authority and PCT over responsibility for the care of a disabled child, but much of the reasoning is also applicable to adults with long-term needs. The child, aged three, had been fitted with a tracheostomy tube in her throat which needed frequent suctioning and adjustment; assistance was also needed to support the child's mother, who was her sole carer. It was accepted that such assistance was properly 'nursing care' and therefore not that which the local authority could provide under s 2 of the Chronically Sick and Disabled Persons Act 1970. Even though the PCT had a duty to provide such care under the NHS Act 1977, this did not crystallise into a specific duty owed to the child or the mother. The PCT had made a proper decision on the hours of care that it felt were needed, weighing up the various elements of the case, and since the child's 'right to life' and the mother's right to family life under the European Convention had not been jeopardised, the court concluded that it should not impose any further requirement on the health care body to allocate resources to this particular case. It appears then that although the courts will (reluctantly) resolve disagreements between health and social care about the limits of their respective statutory duties, they will not quantify for the benefit of individuals the extent to which those duties translate into actual hours of care.

Joint working

Section 47(3)(a) of the NHS and Community Care Act 1990 requires the local authority to notify the relevant health care body if at any time during the carrying out of an assessment for community care services it appears that there may be a health care need. The effect of the notification is to invite them to assist 'to such extent as is reasonable in the circumstances' in the making of the assessment, and the local authority shall 'take into account' any health care services subsequently provided. The Single Assessment Process (SAP) under the NSF for older people (see above, page 12) is predicated on such a flexibility of assessment across organisational and professional boundaries and is of course facilitated by the availability of Health Act flexibilities.

Research into the impact of community care changes on the experience of primary care in the 1990s showed disappointment at the limited nature of resources available and the slowness of social services' responses (Lymbery, 1998). Later reports, looking particularly at mental health services for older people, found conversely that some GPs lacked confidence in the diagnosis of dementia and were slow to access available services (Audit Commission, 2000b, 2002). Being aware of the possible range of community care services from which patients might benefit is not just a professional obligation; it is a legal obligation. Clements (2004) cites the NHS (General Medical Services) Regulations 1992 as authority for the GP's duty to 'arrange for the referral of patients' for the provision of other services under the National Health Service Act 1977. This does not just cover other medical services; it extends to community care services that the local authority may provide under that Act for the prevention of illness, for people suffering from illness and for aftercare services.

NSF for older people

The *NSF for older people* (DH, 2001a) is policy guidance that, although health care-led, addresses itself to both health and social care communities. Although it specifically addresses those medical conditions that are particularly significant for older people – strokes, fall, and mental health problems in old age – it also prioritises equitable treatment for older people and quality of life issues, for example the emphasis on privacy and dignity for older people in general hospital care. Standards within the NSF are aspirational, rather than justiciable. In the absence of substantive legal protection against discrimination on the basis of age, it will continue to be difficult to challenge clinical judgements on the appropriateness of treatment options or quality of care. The courts' reluctance to overturn resource-based decisions means that effective remedies may not be available to challenge rationing decisions or the inadequacy of support available to carers of older people. Particular innovations of the *NSF for older people* are discussed below:

Standard 1	Rooting out age discrimination by basing NHS services on clinical need and preventing social services departments from using age in their eligibility criteria to restrict access to services
Standard 2	Person-centred care to be achieved through SAP and integrated commissioning arrangements
Standard 3	Access to a range of intermediate care services at home or in designated care settings to prevent unnecessary admission to hospital and provide effective rehabilitation
Standard 4	General hospital care that respects privacy and dignity and which is appropriate and specialist
Standard 5	Progress in reducing the incidence of stroke in the population and to ensure prompt access to integrated stroke care services
Standard 6	Objectives to reduce the number of falls that result in serious injury and to ensure effective treatment and rehabilitation
Standard 7	Access to integrated mental health services to ensure effective diagnosis, treatment and support, including support for carers. There is a focus on depression and dementia and recognition of the particular needs of older people from black and minority ethnic communities
Standard 8	The promotion of health and active life expectancy in older people

The *NSF for older people* is part of a 10-year plan. *Next steps in implementing the national service framework for older people* were outlined in 2006 (DH, 2006b). The emphasis is on dignity and human rights, joined-up care and healthy ageing. It is based on consultation with older people, and messages from research. Improving standards in hospital and care homes, improving competence and leadership in the workforce and involving older people as citizens and service users to improve services are seen as key. The Commission for Social Care Inspection (CSCI), in conjunction with the Audit Commission and the Healthcare Commission, has commented sceptically on progress five years into the 10-year plan for the NSF to improve outcomes for people over 50. The report, *Living well in later life* (Audit Commission et al, 2006), found that although progress had been made, improvement in some areas was slow and changes were not consistent across the country. Although more people were being supported to live at home, and age discrimination in policies and eligibility criteria was being addressed, the overall conclusion was that deep-rooted attitudes to ageing in local public services were hampering plans to improve services for older people. Although older people occupy almost two thirds of hospital beds, they continue to be a low priority in both the planning and development of the health service. Also, a lack of shared direction between partner agencies has resulted in services that are fragmented and confusing. Other services, for example public transport, were also not giving priority to the needs of older people, resulting in lack of mobility and social isolation.

Intermediate care

The development of intermediate care is a concept that crosses the primary care/secondary care divide and includes both health and social care provision. Standard 3 of the *NSF for older people* refers to access to a range of intermediate care services at home or in designated care settings to prevent unnecessary admission to hospital and provide effective rehabilitation. LAC (2001)1 (DH, 2001e) sets out guidance on the commissioning of intermediate care services, and defines such services as time-limited (no longer than six weeks and frequently one or two weeks). LAC (2003)14 (DH, 2003b) also provides that any services that form the package of intermediate care must be provided free of charge for six weeks, as must any item of community equipment or minor adaptation to property costing £1,000 or less. Accurate definition of intermediate care services is therefore critical. Paragraph 14 of the 2001 guidance (DH, 2001e) describes eligible service models as: rapid response, as a service designed to prevent avoidable acute admission; hospital at home, which enables investigations and treatment to take place above the level that would normally be provided in primary care; residential rehabilitation, as a short-term programme of therapy and enablement for people whose medical condition has stabilised; supported discharge at home; and day rehabilitation. The King's Fund (2002) has evaluated intermediate care delivered according to a number of different models but the dilemma of whether it is a service to facilitate hospital discharge or to support the reablement of older people is unresolved.

NHS continuing care

The provision of NHS continuing care is a highly contentious area. Guidance titled *Continuing care: NHS and local councils' responsibilities* (DH, 2001f) makes it clear that:

- the setting of care should not be the sole or main determinant of eligibility (that is, continuing care may be in hospital, in a care home or in the community);
- local eligibility criteria should be based on the nature or complexity or intensity or unpredictability of health care needs;
- patients who require palliative care and whose prognosis is that they are likely to die in the very near future should be able to choose to remain in NHS-funded accommodation. Applications of time limits for this care are not appropriate.

Previous guidance on continuing care (DH, 1995b) was reviewed in the *Coughlan* case (*R v North and East Devon Health Authority, ex parte Coughlan* [2000] 1 WLR 622). The case concerned the threatened closure of a NHS unit in which Ms Coughlan, who was severely disabled, was living. Ms Coughlan herself was being re-assessed as needing 'social care' for which she would pay. There the restrictive criteria that the North and East Devon Health Authority applied were held to be ultra vires the NHS Act 1977, and the Court of Appeal confirmed the NHS's responsibility for continuing inpatient care and community health services for people whose primary need is for health care. Also, in that case, the local authority's duty to provide support services under s 21 of the National Assistance Act 1948 was limited to those which were 'incidental or ancillary' to the provision of residential accommodation. As Ms Coughlan's need was primarily a health care need, the NHS remained responsible for her care and could not transfer responsibility to the local authority. The judgment in the *Coughlan* case remains authoritative despite the modification of guidance, and has been applied in subsequent case law, and interpreted in favour of complainants in cases referred to the NHS ombudsman.

Patients who have suffered strokes or who have neurological conditions requiring substantial nursing care and patients with dementia have been accepted as eligible for continuing NHS care. Such care need not be provided in a hospital or nursing home. The Pointon Case (see above, page 46) concluded with the finding that a person with dementia, cared for by their spouse at home, was eligible for NHS continuing care as respite provision. The decision of the ombudsman was critical of assessment tools that were skewed in favour of physical and acute care, and, like earlier decisions, emphasised that the intensity as well as the complexity of nursing needs could lead to eligibility.

Further guidance in 2005 (DH, 2005b) identified patients meeting continuing care eligibility criteria as those who need two or more people and/or the use of lifting and handling equipment to change position; those who cannot make their basic needs for warmth, food or pain relief known; and those who are at high risk of choking in the management of hydration and nutrition. The guidance also applies to complex medication regimes for unstable conditions, including behavioural management. As such the guidance would apply to older people with mental health problems, as well as those with unstable physical conditions. Within the definition of continuing care, Easterbrook (2005) also includes respite health care, specialist health care equipment and specialist transport.

A further significant judgment on continuing care was given in January 2006 by the High Court in *R (Grogan) v Bexley NHS Care Trust* [2006] EWHC 44 (Admin). Mrs Grogan had multiple sclerosis, was a wheelchair user requiring two people for transfer, and had some cognitive impairment. Having been admitted to hospital following a fall, she was transferred to a care home with nursing. Without deciding whether or not Mrs Grogan did in fact meet the criteria for NHS continuing health care, the High Court set aside the Bexley Care Trust's decision that she did not, because the trust did not have in place or apply criteria that properly identified whether her primary need was a health need, as required by the *Coughlan* judgment. Mrs Grogan further submitted that the level of her nursing needs that had been identified in the RNCC medium and high bandings indicated of itself a primary need for health care that should be met by the NHS. Following the judgment, the Department of Health issued interim guidance (DH, 2006c), pending consultation on a combined framework for NHS continuing health care and NHS-funded nursing care. Strategic health authorities were asked to review their policies and procedures and, if necessary, re-assess service users against new criteria. The approach to be taken is described in the guidance as 'the Primary Health Need Approach', and emphasises the primacy of NHS legal duties in this field. It is the totality of the patient's needs that are to be assessed, not only the patient's actual needs for nursing care; the NHS will then be responsible for meeting all assessed care needs, including accommodation. Such an assessment can take place in the community, or in a care home, not necessarily in hospital. This means that high care needs from a multidisciplinary team, for example, physiotherapists, occupational therapists, social workers and therapists, as well as nursing and medical staff, may mean that the patient is eligible for NHS-funded continuing care. By contrast, the RNCC bands apply only to care by a registered nurse that is incidental or ancillary to the provision of accommodation. The guidance also explains the quantitative and qualitative difference between the different bands, but clarifies that those bandings should have no impact on the continuing care eligibility decision. There is a right to an independent review by the strategic health authority of the application of continuing care guidelines or the RNCC to a particular case. Challenges to the guidelines themselves should, however, be pursued through the NHS complaints procedure.

NHS treatment abroad

Under EU law, citizens of member states are entitled to receive services, including medical services, in any country within the EU. The E-112 scheme enables individuals to apply for authorisation to travel abroad for treatment if it is normally provided within the home member state, but cannot be provided without undue delay; the patient will then be reimbursed for costs incurred. In 2004 Yvonne Watts mounted a challenge to the system; she had been diagnosed with osteoarthritis and was in need of a total hip replacement. She travelled to France for her operation, despite the refusal of Bedford PCT to authorise treatment abroad, because she was not a priority case and could have been treated within usual waiting target times.

Mrs Watts challenged the decision before the European Court of Justice (*R (Watts) v Bedford PCT* [2006] All ER (D) 220 (May)). The court held that the absence of a clearly defined procedure for considering applications for treatment outside the UK was contrary to the EC Treaty as it constituted a restriction of the right to equal treatment under Article 49. 'Undue delay' was to be interpreted in terms of Mrs Watts' medical needs and not in terms of her position on a waiting list. In order to restrict access to treatment elsewhere the PCT had to satisfy the test of proportionality and had to set out clearly the criteria on which and the process by which authorisation would be refused.

UK citizens who live permanently abroad have no continuing right to NHS care. However, people over the age of 60 who are still permanently living in the UK may spend up to six months in a European Economic Area country, and up to three months in any other country, without losing their entitlement. UK citizens who live within the EU and Switzerland have the same entitlement to that country's health services as the country's own citizens (Easterbrook, 2005). Visitors to the UK can receive emergency treatment at a GP surgery, compulsory psychiatric treatment and Accident and Emergency Services, but not free inpatient or follow-up outpatient care. Older people seeking to move abroad should bear these limitations in mind (Easterbrook, 2005).

Hospital discharge

Admission to hospital is a crisis for many older people, and three quarters of those admissions are unplanned (Glasby and Littlechild, 2004). Loss of physical function can undermine confidence, and raise anxieties in patients, professionals and families. Admission to hospital is the precipitating factor in 25% of care home admissions (Willcocks et al, 1987). Conducting statutory assessments under s 47 of the NHS and Community Care Act 1990 to facilitate hospital discharge has been identified as the predominant role of hospital social workers (Lymbery, 1998) and even at the inception of community care, agreements on hospital discharge arrangements between the NHS and local authorities were made a prerequisite of local authorities obtaining government funding (McDonald, 2006).

Patients who have sufficient mental capacity can make the decision to discharge themselves; otherwise, the decision is that of the multidisciplinary team, but ultimately of the consultant in charge of the patient's care. However, if the patient may be in need of community care services, the provisions of the Community Care (Delayed Discharges) Act 2003 come into play. This controversial piece of legislation seeks to prompt social services authorities to ensure the rapid discharge of patients from hospital as a response to fears of 'bed blocking' by mainly elderly patients, and its impact on performance indicators within the acute hospital sector. The Act imposes financial penalties on local authorities when the discharge of patients from hospital is delayed for reasons relating to the provision of community care services or services for carers. Liability depends on a complex notification process that begins with the delivery of a 'section 2 notice' by the responsible NHS body to the social services authority within which the patient is ordinarily resident. The notice states that it is considered that it is unlikely to be safe to discharge the patient from hospital unless one or more community care services or carers' services are made available. The duty arises whether or not the patient or carer has been previously assessed. It is the social services authority's responsibility to carry out an assessment and to decide which, if any services, it will make available (s 4(2)). The responsible NHS body must also decide which services it will make available, and will then give notice, under s 5, of a minimum of three days, of its intention to discharge the patient. The liability to make delayed discharge payments on a daily basis applies if has not been possible to discharge the patient because, and only because, the agreed community care or carers' service has not been made available.

The whole process is predicated on medical notions of risk (the 'safe' discharge), rather than social notions of the 'good' discharge in which the patient and carer are fully involved, have time to make choices including that of 'preferred' accommodation (see page 100) and prepare for a planned return home. Supporting guidance, *Discharge from hospital: Pathway, process and practice*, was published by the Department of Health in 2003 (DH, 2003c), which recommends the appointment of 'care coordinators' at ward level and integrated discharge planning teams. These teams would then hold legal responsibility for discharge and patients should be assessed for rehabilitation or eligibility for continuing care before any decisions on alternative care options are made. Lymbery (2005) sees the Community Care (Delayed Discharges) Act 2003 as a catalyst for new thinking on inter-professional working with older people and as an opportunity for real partnership working. To what extent has this hope been realised?

A report by the CSCI (2005) found that decisions made at the time of discharge from hospital can have long-term consequences; very few people who go into residential care at this time return to their own homes, yet they are less likely to need residential care if the right support and rehabilitation is offered to them after leaving hospital. The report calls for a 'genuinely comprehensive preventative approach' for the importance to older people of being cared for by one carer who they know well, for better contingency planning to avoid readmission to hospital, and for a focus on rehabilitation not just administering care. Loneliness, chronic ill health, depression, poverty and feeling unsafe in one's own neighbourhood are major risk factors contributing to the deterioration of health and quality of life in old age. The research concludes that although the system has achieved its objectives for the agencies there continue to be risks within it for vulnerable older people themselves.

The Human Rights Act 1998 is of relevance to precipitate decision making when health care needs have to be balanced against social inclusion. Article 8, the right to respect for privacy and family life, is a qualified right, subject to the test of proportionality justifying interference with the right only to the extent necessary in a democratic society. Mitchell (2006) sees Article 8 as being engaged whenever families and service providers are in dispute about the place to which a vulnerable adult should be discharged following hospital treatment. So, in *R (Gunter) v Southwest Staffordshire PCT* [2005] EWHC 1894 (Admin), the PCT was required to consider again its decision to provide continuing care in a residential setting rather than in the community, having given due weight to an observed improvement in the patient's well-being when able to be close to family at home. Similarly, in *R (Goldsmith) v Wandsworth London Borough Council* [2004] EWCA Civ 1170, the decision to discharge a 95-year-old woman from hospital to a nursing home had been taken without any evidence that the impact of the move on her health had been properly assessed by the local authority, which had relied instead on a medical assessment of her nursing needs from which her daughter had been wrongly excluded. Using human rights arguments may thus challenge the standard agency position that it has the right to determine how eligible needs are to be met.

Palliative care

The NHS end of life care programme (DH, 2003d) is an initiative designed to extend training and develop care pathways so that all adult patients nearing the end of life will have access to high quality specialist palliative care to be able to live and die in the place of their choice. Who provides the service, health or social care, is often not clear. The House of Commons Health Committee report on *Palliative care* (2004) produced a response from government (DH, 2004c) that addresses the following issues:

- The importance of person-centred assessments to address difficulties for patients caused by a focus on personal care within social services to the detriment of equally important domestic support for cleaning and for aids and adaptation.
- Clarification within continuing care guidance that funding should be provided regardless of anticipated life expectancy. Also, that personal care for palliative care patients is the responsibility of the NHS.
- The development of care pathways to meet the risk that the reimbursement system for delayed discharge may have the unintended consequence of treating those in hospice care as a lower priority for discharge to a place of their choice.

Consent to treatment

It is a general principle of common law that consent to medical treatment is required and any action taken without consent amounts to an assault even though no harm may be done. The patient, however, cannot demand treatment that the medical team considers not to be clinically effective (BMA, 2001). An explanation in broad terms of the procedure and its likely effects is sufficient (*Sidaway v Bethlem Royal Hospital Governors* [1985] 1 All ER 643). The decision as to which risks should be disclosed was seen in this case primarily as a matter of clinical judgement in accordance with practice accepted at the time as proper by a responsible body of medical opinion. Generally, disclosure should cover all important risks of the procedure that is proposed, unless such disclosure would cause serious harm to the patient. Only a person who has the capacity to make decisions and who is free of undue influence from others can give consent (Montgomery, 2003). In an emergency situation reliance is placed on the doctrine of necessity to justify intervention without consent, based on the (temporary) incapacity of the patient (see below).

Mental incapacity

The situation of people who are, or are becoming, mentally incapacitated, that is, unable to make decisions for themselves, poses real dilemmas for social workers (Dawson and McDonald, 2000) as well as for doctors. The Mental Capacity Act 2005 seeks to incorporate some of the recommendations of the Law Commission's (1995) enquiry into mental capacity, and to replace the common law with a statutory definition of capacity. It is anticipated that the Act will come into force in April 2007. The key principles contained in the Act are (s 1):

- there is a presumption of capacity;
- individuals must be supported to make their own decisions, as far as it is practicable to do so;
- people are not to be treated as lacking capacity simply because they make unwise decisions;
- everything done for a person lacking capacity is to be done in that person's best interests; a test which has both a social and a medical component;
- the 'least restrictive option' principle must always be considered.

Capacity itself depends on cognitive ability to make decisions (s 2). It comprises the ability to comprehend information relevant to a decision; an ability to remember that information or to believe that information; an ability to weigh in the balance different pieces of information to arrive at a decision; and the ability to communicate that decision (s 3). Some older people may not be able to meet these criteria, or may have a capacity that fluctuates. Capacity, however, is not a global concept; legally it relates to a particular decision, so that there are different and more complex tests of capacity according to the gravity of the decision to be made. Capacity to consent to medical treatment is discussed here and capacity to make a will or to deal with one's financial affairs is dealt with in Chapter Four. Although medical evidence may be sought in these more complex cases, capacity arises as an everyday issue in ordinary transactions where a person refuses medication, or food, or refuses help with personal care (Dawson and McDonald, 2000).

Planning ahead for mental incapacity may be something that older people are reluctant to do. Age Concern produce an excellent fact sheet on advance statements, advance directives and living wills (Age Concern, 2006a) to encourage people to anticipate a time when they may be unable on a temporary or permanent basis to communicate their wishes about medical care. Under the Mental Capacity Act 2005 there are three ways in which decisions may be made concerning future medical treatment:

- Through the creation of an advance decision to refuse treatment (s 24) (see page 68). In the case of life-sustaining treatment, an advance decision is effective only if it is in writing, signed and witnessed.
- Through the creation of a lasting power of attorney (s 9), which authorises in advance another person or persons to make decisions about personal welfare as well as property and business affairs (see page 69).
- Through a decision of the reorganised Court of Protection (s 15), which may make a declaration on the lawfulness of acts done or contemplated, or appoint a person (a 'court appointed deputy') to make such decisions on behalf of the patient.

The patient may in addition nominate a relative or friend as "a person to be consulted in matters affecting his interests" (s 40). What if there is no such person apart from professional or paid carers? Section 35 requires independent mental capacity advocates to be appointed for ascertaining the wishes and feelings of the patient, exploring what alternative courses of action may be available and obtaining a further medical opinion. Such advocates will have access to health records. Any information given by or submissions made by the independent mental capacity advocate must be taken into account when an NHS body is proposing to provide 'serious medical treatment' or long-term accommodation. The decision must then be taken in the patient's best interests. This is an important development to challenge medical opinion and to ensure that the concerns of vulnerable patients are heard.

Advance directives

An advance directive, or 'Living Will', is a means by which an individual may make their wishes known about how they would like to be treated if they become incapable of making a decision for themselves, either because the situation is an emergency and they are unable to communicate or because they have lost capacity due, for example, to dementia or having had a stroke.

An advance directive is a formal means of expressing an intention to refuse some or all forms of medical treatment. It may be verbal or in writing but must cover the specific circumstances which arise. In such cases under common law, medical practitioners are required to follow the patient's wishes, for example to refuse a blood transfusion or an amputation. An advance directive can only be made by a person with mental capacity and is effective only when that person becomes mentally incapacitated. A refusal of basic nursing care or a request for an illegal or medically inappropriate intervention will be ineffective. An advance directive once made should be reviewed by the patient to make sure that it continues to reflect their views in the light of changes in medical treatment.

Sections 24–26 of the Mental Capacity Act 2005 in effect codify the law in this area, using the terminology of "advance decisions to refuse treatment". Such decisions need not be in writing, but will be invalidated by a later lasting power of attorney that gives authority to give or refuse consent to the treatment to which the advance decision relates. The Act places limitations on the effectiveness of advance desisions in a number of ways:

- s 25(4)(c) says that an advance decision is not *valid* if there are reasonable grounds for believing that circumstances exist which the patient did not anticipate and which would have affected their decision;

- an advance decision is not *applicable* to life-sustaining treatment unless it is in writing and witnessed. 'Life sustaining treatment' here could mean emergency surgery or the administration of antibiotics, as well as artificial nutrition and hydration; and
- interim emergency treatment may be given whilst a decision is sought from the Court of Protection on the validity of the advance decision.

Lasting powers of attorney

Section 9 of the Mental Capacity Act 2005 introduces two types of lasting powers of attorney: one for dealing conventionally with "property and affairs"; and a new power to deal with personal welfare issues, which can include (or exclude) health care decisions. An attorney for personal welfare cannot make decisions about the giving or refusal of life-sustaining treatment unless express provision is made (although current proposals simply require a tick-box to this effect to be completed on the prescribed form). The attorney's powers will extend (unless specifically limited) to consent to medical treatment, access to medical records, the provision of community care services, and entry to residential care. Under the law of agency, the attorney has a duty of care to the donor, and is required by s 4 of the Mental Capacity Act 2005 to act in the donor's best interests. The power comes into effect only when the donor becomes mentally incapacitated and the power is registered. In order for the power to be valid, an 'appropriate person' – drawn from a list which includes a registered social worker but which excludes paid carers or managers or employees of care homes in which the donor is living – must certify that the donor understands the purpose of the lasting power and its consequences, and is not acting under undue influence. There is currently no guidance on the level of capacity required to enter into a lasting power of attorney, despite the importance of the decisions being delegated.

Best interest decisions

Section 5 of the Mental Capacity Act 2005 resolves uncertainty about the legal authority of both informal and professional carers by stating that any act in connection with care or treatment performed in the reasonable belief that it is in the patient's best interests will not incur legal liability, except in negligence, if the person giving the care reasonably believes that the patient lacks capacity in relation to the matter. This 'best interests' test is further described in s 4 and, in relation to the principles of equal consideration and non-discrimination, specifically excludes the person's age as an overriding criterion. The decision maker must:

- consider all relevant circumstances;
- consider if and when the person is likely to regain capacity (and thus make the minimum necessary intervention);
- permit and encourage the person to participate in any decision making as far as reasonably practicable;
- ascertain the person's past and present wishes and feelings, and beliefs and values likely to influence his decision
- take into account if practicable and appropriate the views of carers or other persons interested in the patient's welfare.

In the case of life-sustaining treatment, the motivation must not be to bring about the patient's death.

The decision maker is therefore constrained by the need to acknowledge the individuality of the patient. Further guidance to which decision makers must 'have regard' is to be contained in a Code of Practice under the Act, currently under consultation (Department for Constitutional Affairs, 2006).

End of life issues

The decision to stop invasive medical treatment of people at the end of life is a complex one and can arise in both acute and long-term settings. Staff in care homes need to be aware of legal duties as do social workers in hospital settings. Resuscitation, withdrawal of treatment, permanent (or persistent) vegetative state and the right to die are considered here.

Resuscitation

Resuscitation means cardiopulmonary resuscitation (CPR) carried out when a patient's cardiac or respiratory function stops (Easterbrook, 2005). The British Medical Association has set out guidance detailing the circumstances when a DNR (do not resuscitate) decision can be made (BMA, 2002). The decision is that of the consultant in charge of the patient's care. The circumstances are:

- that the patient's condition is such that resuscitation is unlikely to succeed;
- that the patient, having capacity, has made their decision not to be resuscitated in the circumstances that arise;
- that there is a relevant advance directive or living will;
- that resuscitation would not be in the patient's best interest because it would lead to an intolerable quality of life.

Those involved in such decisions should be mindful of the imperative not to discriminate against older people.

Withdrawal of treatment

Medical attendants may legally withdraw treatment when the situation is hopeless. *An NHS Trust v X* [2005] EWCA Civ 1145 concerned an elderly man suffering from chronic renal failure. The trust sought a declaration that invasive treatment should be discontinued and only palliative care given. The key question identified by the Court of Appeal was whether there was any chance of the patient recovering any quality of life so as to justify his continued discomfort. Although the views of his family and religious beliefs (he was a Muslim) had to be taken into account, the court was under a duty to declare that continuing treatment was not in the best interests of the patient on the medical evidence, which showed that there was only a 20%-25% chance of recovery. Avoiding invasive treatment that would not enable the patient to die with dignity was similarly the basis of the best interests declaration in *Portsmouth NHS Trust v Wyatt* [2004] EWHC 2247, where the patient was in a vegetative condition; movements interpreted by family members in that case as signs of responsiveness were attributed to the nature of the patient's condition and not to a hope of recovery.

Permanent vegetative state

The Royal College of Physicians has produced guidance of its own on the diagnosis and management of people in a permanent vegetative state (2003). Key to the diagnosis (para 3.5) is that recovery cannot reasonably be expected, and further therapy is futile. The diagnosis should be discussed sensitively with relatives who should be given time to consider the implications, including the possibility of withdrawing artificial means of administering nutrition and hydration. At present in England and Wales the courts require that disputes over the decision to withdraw nutrition and hydration (although not to commence it) should be referred to them before any action is taken (Montgomery, 2003). The Royal College's checklist requires six months to have elapsed since the onset of the vegetative state before it is diagnosed as permanent (one year in the case of head injury), and specifies professionals who are to be involved in the decision, and the clinical tests that have to be carried out. Disagreement between family members is pre-empted by the statement (in Appendix 1) that the continuing disagreement of one individual with the conclusion of health professionals and others close to the patient is not a bar to the diagnosis of the vegetative state.

The leading case is *Airedale NHS Trust v Bland* [1993] 1 All ER 821, which concerned a survivor of the Hillsborough Football Stadium disaster who remained in a persistent vegetative state, although he did not require mechanical life support. Doctors wanted to withdraw artificial feeding and hydration, and the House of Lords granted a declaration that this would not be unlawful, having rejected any distinction between the provision of food and water and other aspects of care which might be withdrawn (Montgomery, 2003). It appears that the law on withholding or withdrawing life-sustaining treatment has not been altered by the Human Rights Act 1998. In *An NHS Trust v M; An NHS Trust v H* [2001] 2 FLR 367, it was held that a decision to withdraw treatment was not an intentional deprivation of life under Article 2; furthermore, reliance was placed on the *Bolam* test (see page 88) to say that where a responsible body of medical opinion led to a clinical decision that it was not in the best interests of a patient to prolong treatment, then the positive obligation on the state to take reasonable steps to preserve life had been discharged (Montgomery, 2003).

Right to die

A challenge to the power of the medical establishment to make life or death decisions was made in *R (Burke) v GMC* [2005] EWCA Civ 1003 by a disabled man who wanted assurance that his life would not be prematurely ended. It was held that the guidance to doctors on withholding and withdrawing life-prolonging treatment (GMC, 2002) did not infringe Articles 2, 3 or 8 of the European Convention on Human Rights because it recognised that artificial nutrition and hydrocation could not be withdrawn before the final stages of life and by doing so it was in accordance with the decision of the House of Lords in the *Bland* case. The Court of Appeal in the *Burke* case interestingly refused to become involved in responding to a request for a wide-ranging declaration on issues that they described as "fundamentally important questions of medical law and ethics", but did acknowledge that the threshold of intolerable quality of life was the proper boundary for the withdrawal of medical treatment.

It had already been established in the case of Diane Pretty, both in the House of Lords (*Pretty v DPP* [2002] 1 All ER 1) and the European Court of Human Rights (*Pretty v UK* [2002] 2 FCR 97) that in the converse situation, the 'right to life' (Article 2) did not include the 'right to die' by means of assisted suicide. The right of a mentally competent patient to refuse life-prolonging treatment was, however, reiterated in the case of Miss B (*Re B (Consent to Treatment: Capacity)* [2002] All ER 429) where the patient made the decision against medical advice. Anxieties about the limits of social services' responsibility were addressed in the case of Z (*Re Z (Local Authority: Duty)* [2005] 1 WLR 959), who informed staff of her intention to go abroad to seek assisted suicide. The High Court refused to continue an injunction granted to the local authority who were providing services to the woman in her own home. The extent of their duty was to inform the police if they felt any criminal act was likely to be committed and to alert the court to any concerns about her capacity, but otherwise the local authority (and the court) could do nothing. The court was specifically concerned in that case to protect the right of a progressively ill person to take autonomous decisions in the face of professional anxiety.

Parliament has responded to demands for legislation in this complex area through the Assisted Dying for the Terminally Ill Bill (defeated in Parliament in May 2006). The Bill would have made it lawful for a physician to assist the death of a patient who has a terminal illness and who makes a written request to die. No assistance could have been given where a consultant psychiatrist or psychologist determined that the patient lacked capacity. That situation remains to be determined by common law or the application of the Mental Capacity Act 2005 (see above).

Mental health

Services for older people with mental health problems have similarities with and differences from services for younger people. In the Audit Commission's research into services for older people (2000b), specialist help for users and carers was found to be patchy and uncoordinated. Person-centred approaches require considerable resources and skill to put into practice (Innes et al, 2006). One quarter of those over the age of 85 will develop dementia, with one third of this group requiring constant care or supervision. Depression is also common among older people, affecting between 10% and 16% of those over 65; more than this when the population in residential care is considered. A useful and updated practice guide has been produced by the Social Care Institute for Excellence, *Assessing the mental health needs of older people* (SCIE, 2006), which covers policy and guidance, an overview of current practice, the Mental Health Act 1983 and older people and the needs of black and minority ethnic groups.

Care Programme Approach

The Department of Health has clarified the relationship between SAP and the specialist Care Programme Approach (CPA) for people referred to secondary psychiatric assessment and has addressed issues of transition (DH, 2002d). Older people with psychotic illness, for example schizophrenia, should, according to the guidance, be on CPA, but the assessment of their needs should be based on SAP for older people. The CPA process should also be applied to other older people with severe functional or organic mental health problems who, if they were younger, would be provided for under CPA. When individuals subject to CPA reach transition age, movement on from it should only be made in the best interests of individuals and should ensure continuity of care.

Because the incidence of mental disorder may be associated with bereavement or changes in lifestyle, legal mechanisms need to be sensitive to the varying needs of people at different stages of their illness; this is particularly so with dementia, which is a progressive disorder. Care must be taken, however, not to exclude people with community care needs from services because they do not meet CPA criteria of having severe and enduring mental illness. So, in *R (HP and KP) v Islington London Borough Council* [2004] EWHC 7 (Admin), Munby J required the local authority to reassess the needs of an elderly man suffering from reactive depression and possibly in the early stages of dementia; he was at risk of self-neglect and a deterioration in his mental state although he did not meet CPA criteria. There was still, however, a duty to assess his need for community care services under s 47 of the NHS and Community Care Act 1990. CPA is thus not the only way into services for people with mental health problems in the community. When the offer of services is refused, giving cause for concern for the patient's welfare, the exercise of compulsion may need to be considered.

Mental Health Act 1983

The current legislation is the Mental Health Act 1983, supported by the Memorandum under the Act, and the 1999 Code of Practice. The opening paragraph of the Code of Practice (DH, 1999) explains how the principles of the Mental Health Act should be put into practice. People to whom the Act applies (including those being assessed for possible admission to hospital) should:

• receive recognition of their basic human rights under the European Convention on Human Rights;
• be given respect for their qualities, abilities and diverse backgrounds as individuals and be assured that account will be taken of their age, gender, sexual orientation, social, ethnic, cultural and religious backgrounds, but that general assumptions will not be made on the basis of any one of those characteristics;
• have their needs taken fully into account, although it is recognised that, within available resources, it may not always be practicable to meet them in full;
• be given any necessary treatment or care in the least controlled and segregated facilities compatible with ensuring their own health and safety or the safety of other people;
• be treated and cared for in such a way as to promote to the greatest practicable degree their self-determination and personal responsibility, consistent with their own needs and wishes;
• be discharged from detention or other powers provided by the Act as soon as it is clear that their application is no longer justified.

Although the Code of Practice has the status of guidance, good and cogent reasons have to be given for a departure from its requirements, either in relation to individual patients or identifiable classes of patients (*R v Ashworth Hospital Authority ex parte Munjaz* [2005] UKHL 58). In fact a number of the provisions of the Mental Health Act 1983 and of common law have been challenged for their incompatibility with the European Convention on Human Rights, and this will need to be reflected in any proposed changes to legislation in this field.

The Mental Health Act itself sets out those circumstances in which compulsory admission to hospital for assessment and treatment may be authorised. Much of the Act is based on the exercise of professional discretion. The professionals concerned are registered medical practitioners "authorised as having special training in the assessment and treatment of mental disorder" (s 12); these are consultant psychiatrists and also some GPs. Approved social workers are appointed by the local authority to introduce a social element into the assessment, but operate as independent practitioners.

Section 131 of the Act, however, makes it clear that, for anyone over the age of 16 and capable of expressing their own wishes, informal admission should be the norm. The term used is 'informal', not 'voluntary' admission, the emphasis thus being on an absence of resistance rather than a positive giving of consent. This has proved controversial in the case of mentally incapacitated patients, as will be seen. The majority of admissions are in fact informal, particularly in the case of older people (DH, 2005c). Informal admission may avoid conflict and possibly stigma. Arguably it can also have the effect of depriving patients of their civil rights under this Act and under the European Convention on Human Rights.

Nearest relative

In all cases application for admission (based on medical recommendation) can be made either by an approved social worker or by the patient's nearest relative. This process is commonly known as 'sectioning'. Most applications are by an approved social worker, but s 26 of the Mental Health Act 1983 itself provides a hierarchy for deciding who is the nearest relative in any case. This hierarchy is:

> Husband or wife of the patient (including cohabitees who have lived with the patient for more than six months)
> Son or daughter
> Father or mother
> Brother or sister
> Grandparent
> Grandchild
> Uncle or aunt
> Niece or nephew

The nearest relative is the person first described in this list, with the eldest in any category taking precedence, regardless of sex. However, where the patient ordinarily resides with or is cared for by one of their relatives, that relative shall be given preference over any other.

The European Court of Human Rights in *JT v UK* [2000] 1

FLR 909 has held that the rigid application of s 26 is contrary to Article 8 of the European Convention on Human Rights when it has the effect of enabling a relative from whom the patient is estranged to make decisions relating to the patient's private affairs. Also, the wording of s 26 appears to exclude same-sex partners from being nearest relatives. A solution to both of these situations has been found by interpretation by the courts without the need for a declaration of incompatibility or formal amendment to date of the Mental Health Act. So, in *R (on the application of SSG) v Liverpool City Council and Secretary of State for Health (CO/1220/ 2002)*, a Consent Order was made declaring that the same-sex partner of a patient could be treated as falling within the phrase "living with the patient as the patient's husband or wife as the case may be" in s 26(6). The need to protect the patient's Article 8 rights by not notifying their nearest relative of the application for detention has been protected by interpreting the term 'practicable' under s 22 so as to excuse the approved social worker from informing (s 2) or consulting with (s 3) the nearest relative, taking into account the patient's wishes and their health and well-being (*R (on the application of E) v Bristol City Council* [2005] All ER (D) 57). The Department of Health has subsequently accepted that the guidance given in paragraph 2.16 of the Code of Practice that "Practicality refers to the availability of the nearest relative and not to the appropriateness of informing or consulting the person concerned" is no longer correct, although approved social workers should not lightly invoke their power to exclude people, particularly as s 29 enables the nearest relative who acts unreasonably to be displaced by application to the county court.

Mental disorder

Central to the functioning of the Mental Health Act 1983 is the definition of 'mental disorder' in s 1(2). There are four specific forms of mental disorder: mental illness; arrested or incomplete development of mind; psychopathic disorder and 'any other disorder of disability of mind'. The inclusion of 'arrested or incomplete development of mind' within the definition of mental disorder means that people with learning difficulties may come within some sections of the Mental Health Act 1983. Promiscuity or other immoral conduct, sexual deviancy, or dependence on drugs or alcohol do not in themselves constitute a mental disorder (s 1(3) Mental Health Act 1983). Mental illness is nowhere defined in the Act, nor have the courts given any real guidance as to its proper interpretation; its meaning therefore is a matter of clinical practice. Reference may be made to SCIE guidance (SCIE, 2006) for definitions and procedures relating to the admission of older people.

Admission for assessment

The grounds for admission under s 2 of the Mental Health Act 1983 are that the patient is suffering from mental disorder of a nature or degree that warrants their detention in a hospital for assessment (or for assessment followed by medical treatment) for a limited period of up to 28 days. An application for admission must be founded on the written recommendations of two medical practitioners, one of whom must be approved as having special experience in the diagnosis and treatment of mental disorder and one of whom should, if practicable, have had previous acquaintance with the patient. The applicant must have personally seen the patient within the previous 14 days and admission must take place within 14 days of the date of the second medical examination. Section 2 of the Mental Health Act 1983 is appropriate where the patient is unknown to services or the diagnosis is unclear.

Section 4 contains a provision for emergency admission for assessment on the grounds that it is of urgent necessity for the patient to be admitted and detained under s 2 (above), but that compliance with all the procedural formalities would involve undesirable delay. Only one medical recommendation is needed and the doctor need not be approved; however, he should, if practicable, have had previous acquaintance with the patient and must have seen them within the previous 24 hours from the time of admission to hospital. The authority to detain lapses after 72 hours unless it is 'converted' to a s 2 admission by the giving of a second medical recommendation. There is no formal power of discharge or appeal in respect of emergency admission for assessment. It is of concern that in some cases s 4 powers may be open to abuse by being applied in non-emergency situations.

Admission for treatment

Admission for treatment under s 3 of the 1983 Act is a far more draconian power than admission for assessment since it involves the power to give treatment to a patient (subject to some limitations) without their consent. The period of detention is also longer, being for an initial (but renewable) period of up to six months. Such an application cannot be made by an approved social worker if the nearest relative (who should in any case be consulted) objects. An application for admission must be founded on the written recommendations of two medical practitioners. The classes of people liable to be detained under s 3 are also more limited. The patient must be suffering from mental illness, psychopathic disorder, severe mental impairment or mental impairment. Severe mental impairment and mental impairment must, however, be associated with 'abnormally aggressive or seriously irresponsible conduct'. There is also a 'treatability' test in the case of psychopathic disorder or mental impairment; that is, the treatment to be given on admission should be such as is likely to alleviate or prevent a deterioration in their condition.

Powers of entry and powers of detention

There may be circumstances in which entry to premises is being refused and legal powers need to be sought. These are contained in s 115 and s 135 of the Act.

Section 115 authorises an approved social worker to enter and inspect any premises that are not a hospital and in which a mentally disordered patient is living if they have reasonable cause to believe that the patient is not under proper care. It is an offence for anyone to obstruct them without reasonable cause (s 129). Section 115, however, does not permit entry by force, nor does it contain any power of removal. For these latter purposes, a warrant under s 135 of the Act authorising a police constable to make entry is needed.

Section 115 and s 135 deal with people found on private premises. However, s 136 gives the police power to detain people "who appear to be suffering from mental disorder and to be in immediate need of care and control" who are found in places "to which the public have access". Removal is to a 'place of safety', but must be "either in the interests of the person concerned or necessary for the protection of other people". No central records are kept of the use of this section but obviously the 72-hour period of detention authorised by s 136 is capable of being used for *de facto* admission if the police take the patient directly to hospital.

Admission of mentally incapacitated patients

The '*Bournewood* gap' has exposed a hiatus in the application of the Mental Health Act 1983 to protect people who are mentally incapacitated. Relying on the common law doctrine of necessity, the House of Lords in *R v Bournewood Community and Mental Health NHS Trust ex parte L* [1999] 1 WLR 107 declared not unlawful the admission to hospital of L, who was autistic and unable to consent to his admission, but made no attempt to leave. His situation would be paralleled by that of many older people with cognitive impairments. Reliance on common law, enabling the formal processes of the Mental Health Act 1983 to be bypassed, was a source of concern, not least to L's carers, who challenged the conformity of his admission with the European Convention before the European Court of Human Rights. The European Court (*HL v UK* (2004) 40 EHRR 761) found that L was unlawfully detained, dismissing the argument that he was free to leave at any time. The absence of a clear and generally known process for his detention contravened Article 5. His inability to challenge his detention also amounted to a breach of Article 5(4).

The Department of Health (DH, 2005c) has provided guidance on the findings and implications of the European Court of Human Rights judgment in the *Bournewood* case (*HL v UK* (above)). The guidance acknowledges that the judgment could extend to other groups of people 'of unsound mind' within Article 5 who are deprived of their liberty in hospital, and perhaps also to similar people in non-hospital settings such as care homes. Deprivation of liberty could also include control through medication or preventing people from leaving due to physical frailty or the locking of doors on open units. The decision for which capacity would need to be lacking in the *Bournewood* context is that the person is not capable of consenting to such constraints as amount to a deprivation of liberty. But, as the guidance shows, there is no clear threshold at which restrictions placed on different freedoms of choice amount to an overall deprivation of liberty such as freedom of movement, contact with visitors or choice of treatment.

Complex cases funding

Patients with complex needs whose mental health has stabilised following the acute phase and who may be seeking rehabilitation elsewhere are often referred to funding panels for placement. One issue then is the extent to which such a panel is required to accept a recommendation for transfer, often done by way of s 17 leave while the patient continues to be compulsorily detained. Some clarification of this issue was introduced by *R (K) v West London Mental Health*

NHS Trust [2006] EWCA Civ 118, which concerned a patient at Broadmoor Hospital who was recommended for transfer to a medium-security hospital in the private sector by his responsible medical officer. Although the officer had the right under the Mental Health Act 1983 to make the decision, it was held that it was open to the PCT funding the patient to refuse to fund the transfer either on the grounds of clinical judgement or resource considerations. A panel decision enabled the views of others properly to be taken into account and to establish priorities. The judgment therefore is an interesting one in moving towards collective decision making even where legislation allocates decision making to individuals or other bodies (in this case a mental health review tribunal had supported the plan). The absence of a statutory duty on the organisation to facilitate those decisions means that resources cannot compulsorily be allocated to support it. Patients then may lawfully remain in hospital when funding is not available for community support.

Guardianship

Guardianship is a legal device whereby a degree of formal control can be exercised over people who are suffering from mental disorder but who remain within the community or who are to be discharged to the community. Its best use is in a supportive way to enable the provision of services which might otherwise be refused (Mitchell, 2006). Guardianship might also be used, within Chapter 17 of the Code of Practice, when elderly people in residential care are expressing a wish to leave in circumstances in which this would not be in their own best interests and informal persuasion is inadequate.

The grounds for reception into guardianship in civil cases are contained in s 7(1) of the Mental Health Act 1983. The patient must be suffering from mental illness, psychopathic disorder, severe mental impairment or mental impairment of a nature or degree that warrants their reception into guardianship and it must be necessary in the interests of the welfare of the patient or for the protection of other people that the patient should be so received. In contrast to the Mental Health Act 1959, which gave the guardian all the powers that a parent has over a child under the age of 14, the Mental Health Act 1983 limits the powers of the guardian to three particular instances:

1. to require the patient to reside at a place specified by the guardian;

2. to require the patient to attend for medical treatment, education or training; and
3. to require access to the patient to be given to any doctor, approved social worker or any other person similarly specified (s 8(2)).

It is the limited nature of these powers and the lack of any sanctions for their breach that is the main reason for guardianship's lack of popularity (in the year ending March 2005 there were 932 cases open, but 10% of all local authorities accounted for 43% of cases).

A private individual may be appointed guardian, but they must have the approval of their local social services authority so to act; in the majority of cases it will be the local authority that is appointed guardian. Guardianship lasts for an initial period of six months but may be renewed for a further six months and then for a year at a time. The local authority has visiting duties during the period of guardianship. It is particularly important to note that guardianship gives no authority over financial affairs; for that, a separate application should be made to the Court of Protection (see Chapter Four).

Mental health review tribunals

Mental health review tribunals incorporate a quasi-judicial element into the law of mental health by providing a means by which appeal can be made against compulsory detention or the imposition of guardianship. Patients admitted for assessment can apply within the first 14 days of their admission and patients admitted for treatment or received into guardianship can apply during the first six months. There is also a procedure for the automatic review of all patients admitted for treatment under civil powers who have not exercised their right to apply within the first six months. Further reviews will be carried out at intervals of not less than three years.

There is a tribunal for each of the separate health authority regions comprising a legal chair, a medical member and a layperson. The tribunal must sit in private to take evidence (unless the patient asks for it to be in public), usually at the hospital at which the patient is detained. There is no appeal from the decision of a mental health review tribunal, although, if a misinterpretation of its powers or procedural impropriety is alleged, there is the possibility of judicial review in the High Court.

Conflicts between mental health review tribunal procedures and the European Convention on Human Rights have led to Declarations of Incompatibility under the Human Rights Act 1998, leading to a change in the burden of proof in s 72 of the Mental Health Act 1983 so that it became necessary for the detaining authority to prove that the patient's mental condition warranted their continuing detention, and changes in the listing of cases for hearing by tribunals to avoid unreasonable delay. In *R (H) v Secretary of State for Health* [2005] All ER (D) 218, s 2 of the Mental Health Act 1983 was considered for its compatibility with Article 5 of the European Convention based on the impracticability of an incapacitated patient being able to challenge their detention during the 28-day time limit when proceedings had been brought under s 29 to displace the nearest relative. The House of Lords, reversing the decision of the Court of Appeal, held that the difficulties that the patient, who had Downs syndrome, would face in taking proceedings to challenge her detention did not of itself make Article 2 incompatible with the Convention, although the inaction of the authorities might make it so. However, if the court came to a speedy decision on the displacement of the nearest relative or the Secretary of State used their power to refer the case to a tribunal, this would provide an adequate means of redress. There were also other remedies available though habeas corpus and judicial review.

Aftercare duties

Section 117 of the Mental Health Act 1983 imposes a duty on health and social services authorities to provide 'aftercare' services for those who have been detained for treatment. Aftercare services are 'community care services' under the definition in s 46(3) of the NHS and Community Care Act 1990. This is a specific statutory duty, narrower in its scope than the provision of aftercare under CPA. The only patients eligible under s 117 are those detained under s 3 for treatment, s 37 by order of a criminal court and ss 47 and 48 on transfer from prison on remand to hospital on the Order of the Home Secretary. While there is no restriction on the type of services that can be provided under s 117 aftercare, it is not a 'gateway' to other statutory services. Services provided under s 117 cannot be charged for (*R v Manchester County Council ex parte Stennett and others* [2002] 3 WLR 584). It is important therefore to ascertain under what statutory power a particular service is being provided: in the *Stennett* case, the local authority argued that the applicant's residential care was provided (as would be usual) under s 21 of the National Assistance Act 1948, to which charges would be applied. The House of Lords decided, however, that the care was provided under s 117, with the consequence that substantial numbers of claims were made for reimbursement.

The extent of the duty under s 117 to find residential accommodation was considered by the local government ombudsman in a case involving York City Council (04/B/1280) (cited in Mitchell, 2006). The family of an elderly patient detained under s 3 were left to find her a residential placement. Although the local authority's duty was only to use its 'best endeavours' (*R (B) v Camden London Borough Council* [2005] EWHC 1366 (Admin)) to find a placement, there was nothing so unusual about the circumstances of this older person's case that prevented a delay of 12 months in securing accommodation from being maladministration. The ombudsman also saw the s 117 duty as arising prior to discharge when it was apparent that residential care was needed following the failure of a trial at home.

The duty to provide aftercare services is placed jointly on the health and social services authority for the area in which the patient was resident at the time they were detained. Services must be provided until the authorities jointly decide (probably by means of a CPA meeting) that the patient is no longer in need of such services. The patients themselves, and their relatives, should be parties to this decision. Discharge from the consultant's list may not of itself determine the end of the s 117 duty. The duration of the duty in respect of people with dementia was considered in *R v Richmond London Borough Council and others ex parte Watson* [2001] 1 All ER 436. Sullivan J held that:

> There may be cases where, in due course there will be no more need for aftercare services for the person's mental condition but he or she will still need social services provision for other needs, for example, physical disability. Such cases will have to be examined individually on their facts, through the assessment process provided for by s 47 (National Health Service and Community Care Act 1990). In a case … where the illness is dementia, it is difficult to see how such a situation could arise.

The local government ombudsman, in response to the *Stennett* case (above), published a special report in July 2003 because of the number of complaints that had been made of local authorities charging for aftercare when they should not have done so. Social services authorities were asked to put into place arrangements to identify people improperly charged for services and to make restitution to themselves or their estate. The specific cases related to older people whose aftercare had consisted of a permanent placement in a care home. It was held that such placements were to be funded by the local social services/health authority and not the individual. While aftercare is being provided under s 117, the older person in receipt of this will not be eligible for 'needs-tested' benefits from the Department for Work and Pensions, such as Attendance Allowance.

This can give rise to the anomaly that two people suffering similar psychiatric conditions can be admitted to hospital on the same day, one under compulsory section, one informally, and then discharged into the same care home. The one discharged under s 117 of the Mental Health Act 1983 will have fees fully paid for; the 'informal' patient will have to self-fund their home care costs. In reaching its decision, the House of Lords recognised this, but considered that s 117 intended this result – the compulsorily detained person being more vulnerable – which caused the section to be imposed in the first place.

Aftercare in the community was not considered and has not been statutorily defined. It has been considered in the case of *Christopher Clunis v Camden and Islington Health Authority* [1998] 3 All ER 180, where Baldwin LJ described it as normally including:

> ... social work support in helping the ex-patient with problems of employment, accommodation and family relationships, the provision of domiciliary services, and the use of day centre and recreational facilities....

The House of Lords in the *Stennett* case approved the description.

Reform of the Mental Health Act 1983

Following the recommendations of the Richardson Committee (Richardson, 1999), a series of proposals have been put forward to reform the Mental Health Act 1983. These have proved controversial insofar as they cover a wide definition of mental disorder, preventive detention for people with anti-social personality disorder, compulsory treatment in the community and the replacement of the nearest relative, and of the approved social worker.

On 23 March 2006, the Secretary of State for Health announced that instead of introducing a major new Mental Health Act, a shorter streamlined Bill would amend the 1983 Act "to promote patient safeguards and to protect patients and the public from harm". It is anticipated that the Bill will:

- replace the current four categories of mental disorder with a wider definition;
- keep the exclusion for drug and alcohol dependency, but preserve the effect of the Act in relation to people with learning difficulties who display abnormally aggressive or seriously irresponsible conduct;
- replace the current 'treatability' test for patients with psychopathic disorder and mental impairment, with a test applying to all compulsorily detained patients that 'appropriate', if not therapeutic, treatment must be available;
- amend the current provisions on nearest relative in line with the European Convention on Human Rights by widening the range of people who can apply to the court for displacement, and modernising the law in line with the Civil Partnership Act 2004;
- introduce supervised treatment in the community, but only after an initial period of detention and treatment in hospital, enabling recall to hospital if people refuse treatment.

In addition:

- following public consultation on the *Bournewood* case, an amendment will be made to the Mental Capacity Act 2005 for people who lack capacity and are subject to deprivation of liberty, by introducing a clearer procedure prescribed by law in line with the European Convention on Human Rights;
- the safeguard of advocacy for all compelled patients has, however, been removed from the Mental Health Bill as has the proposal for a tribunal to authorise any detention beyond an initial period of 28 days;
- in terms of personnel, the responsible medical officer will be replaced by a clinical supervisor, and the replacement of the approved social worker by an 'approved mental health professional' is retained from earlier Bills;
- the link between renewal of detention and referral for a tribunal hearing will be broken to enable more flexible referrals to take place.

It is likely that these changes will be introduced from 2008.

Challenging health care decisions

Challenging health care decisions may arise in a number of different circumstances: where health and social work agencies dispute responsibility for providing services; where members of a multidisciplinary team disagree; and where patients challenge the quantity or quality of service received.

What is apparent is that even where there is a clear NHS responsibility, for example in the provision of community nursing, social care agencies cannot, through their own assessment processes, compel performance of that duty by health care bodies (*R (D) v Haringey London Borough Council*) (see above, page 56). Professionals working in a multidisciplinary team are legally responsible for their own decisions, although their employer will be vicariously liable for decisions of the whole team, if it is a single employer (such as a partnership trust) (Montgomery, 2003). Members of the team are entitled to rely on the professional judgement of others, although they may need to seek confirmation of decisions or refuse, as a matter of their own professional discretion, to act where mistakes are "grossly obvious" (Montgomery, 2003, p 179). Conversely, the employer is responsible for the provision of adequate support to do the job properly; so, in *Jones v Manchester Corporation* [1952] 2 All ER 125, the employer was liable for providing inadequate supervision for a junior doctor who had made mistakes.

The standard of care required from all health professionals to avoid an action in negligence has been long established as that set out in *Bolam v Friern Hospital* [1957] 2 All ER 118; it is to act "in accordance with a practice accepted as proper by a responsible body of medical men skilled in that particular art". As Montgomery (2003, p 177) comments, "a general practitioner may therefore fail correctly to diagnose a patient's condition without being negligent even though a specialist's failure to make an accurate diagnosis of the same patient would not be acceptable". For social workers, adherence to the General Social Care Council's *Code of practice for social care workers* (2002) would be a minimum requirement for reaching that professional standard. Acting in accordance with agency policies and procedures will not, however, replace scrutiny of professional discretion or compliance with legal duties required by statute (Montgomery, 2003; Braye and Preston-Shoot, 2005).

The National Patient Safety Agency (www.npsa.nhs.uk) has developed policy (2005) to promote better communication between staff and patients when medical treatment goes wrong, recognising that a lack of apology and defensive responses may compound the original injury.

Complaints procedures within the NHS prior to July 2004 were subject to an informal stage of local resolution followed by a request to a complaints convenor (a non-executive director of the trust) for an independent review. Dissatisfactions concerning independence or delays (DH, 2004d) led to changes of procedure in the Health and Social Care (Community Health and Standards) Act 2003. The Healthcare Commission has been given responsibility for undertaking reviews of complaints that are outstanding after local resolution and independent review panel procedures have been undertaken. Where complaints involve different aspects of care such as a PCT, NHS trust or ambulance trust, the Commission will be able to look at the whole of the patient's experience. Patient forums represent consumer interests on health care bodies, and the Patient Advice and Liaison Service (PALS) performs an advocacy role in supporting patients in dispute with services. The health service ombudsman will also consider disputes that cannot be resolved through this process. The NHS Litigation Authority is a special health authority responsible for handling negligence claims against the NHS.

Case study 2: Hospital discharge

Vera Gawlinski is 85 years old. She came to England from Poland in 1946, where she married and had one daughter, Julia. Vera's husband Thomas died two years ago. Since then Vera has lived alone; her daughter lives 200 miles away. Vera has been supported by home care services since her husband died; recently carers have been concerned that Vera is not eating and is neglecting her personal care. She is increasingly forgetful and has recently been diagnosed with dementia. Following an incident when she left a pan on the stove, causing a fire, Vera was admitted to hospital suffering from the effects of smoke inhalation. Julia is concerned that Vera should be given assistance to manage at home when she is discharged from hospital, but is concerned that her mother will neglect to take her medication and that she has lost some confidence during her time in hospital. The time is approaching when Vera will be discharged.

How can the law ensure that Vera's discharge is well planned, and that Vera and her daughter are involved in decisions concerning her future care?

What are the respective responsibilities in this case of health and social care agencies?

Further reading

Glasby, J. and Littlechild, P. (2004) *The health and social care divide*, Bristol: The Policy Press.
Explains the modernising agenda within the NHS, and contains excellent material on hospital discharge and continuing care policy in particular.

Ham, C. (2004) *Health policy in Britain: The politics and organisation of the National Health Service* (5th edn), Basingstoke: Macmillan.
This is a classic text on the history of the NHS, its funding and policies. The fifth edition also contains chapters on health policy in Scotland, Wales and Northern Ireland.

Bartlett, P. and Sandland, R. (2003) *Mental health law: Policy and practice* (2nd edn), Oxford: Oxford University Press.
An accessible and clearly written account of mental health law and practice, which focuses on the concerns of practitioners.

THREE

Housing and residential care

Housing

People's housing needs will be very particular to them as individuals, and a wide range of housing options are therefore necessary to accommodate older people. 'Home' to older people means more than bricks and mortar; it provides a sense of security and identity, particularly if there is continuity over time (Peace et al, 1997). There is a large unmet need for housing repairs and adaptations for older people, who are the group most likely to live in substandard housing (Oldman, 2000). There is also much 'hidden' homelessness among older people who may be occupying property that is not suitable for their needs, and among younger older people who may have mental health problems or a history of substance misuse (SEU, 2006).

Owner-occupation

The growth in home ownership has had an impact on older people in a number of ways. Redundancy and early retirement will mean that one third of owner-occupiers aged 65-74 in 2011 will still have a mortgage to pay (SEU, 2006). Pension Credit can help with payment of interest on loans of £100,000 or less, but this may still mean that people need to free up equity in the property to meet the costs of day-to-day living. There will also be a tension between using capital to pay for care charges (including a move to residential care) and the inheritance expectations of the next generation. This was an issue discussed but not resolved by the Royal Commission on Long-term Care (1999), whose recommendation of free personal care in whatever setting it is needed was taken up in Scotland but not in England and Wales. It was also the focus of the Wanless report (Wanless, 2006), currently under scrutiny by government.

Tenancies in the public and private sector

For those who wish to rent rather than buy there is a mixed economy of provision. Tenancies in the public and private sector may be one of three types, with varying degrees of security of tenure:

- regulated (secure tenancies): granted up to 15 January 1989
- assured tenancies: granted after 15 January 1989
- assured shorthold tenancies: granted after 28 February 1997.

Often specialising in 'special needs' provision, housing associations also take nominations from the local authority's housing register. Almost all local authority or housing association tenancies are secure assured tenancies, which means that there are restricted grounds on which the landlord can seek possession, namely, breach of the tenancy agreement or causing a nuisance to neighbours. By contrast, assured shorthold tenancies in the private sector granted after 28 February 1997 are of six months' duration, with the landlord having a right of possession without giving reasons after two months' notice. In all cases, however, possession cannot be given without a court order, and tenants are protected from harassment under the Prevention of Eviction Act 1977.

Older tenants may be concerned about the right of other family members to succeed to a tenancy on their death. In fact, there are automatic rights of succession for a husband and wife or partner (of either sex) and for other members of the family, provided those other family members have been living with the tenant for a minimum period of two years. However, council tenants may be requested to move to other suitable alternative accommodation if either the home is specifically designed or adapted for someone with a disability, or the home is larger than is needed by the person who has taken over the tenancy.

The 'Right to Buy', which was introduced for local authority tenants in 1980, is restricted to those who have been public sector tenants for a minimum of two years. Some or all of the discount for which buyers are eligible is repayable if the home is sold within three years of purchase. Combinations of renting and purchasing property under shared ownership are possible, whereby the landlord retains a share in the property until such time as the tenant is able to buy them out. Paragraph 11 of Schedule 5 of the Housing Act 1985 places restrictions on the Right to Buy if the property was either let for occupation by a person aged 60 or over, or is particularly suitable for occupation by an older person taking into account its location, size, accessibility and heating systems, ignoring features put in by the tenant. There is a right of appeal to a residential property tribunal following the exclusion of a property from the Right to Buy on these grounds (Cafferkey, 2005).

Supported housing

Sheltered or supported housing schemes may exist in either the private or the public sector, and may be available to buy or to rent. Support may range from on- or off-site warden provision to very sheltered housing schemes where personal and domestic care as well as housing is provided. Supporting People funding (see page 94) may be available to meet the cost of warden services and emergency call systems. A community care assessment may lead to the provision of personal care services, sometimes within a 'package' of housing and social care. Assistive technology, such as fall detectors and videophones, may also be used to enable people to live independently in the community with greater privacy and dignity. The legal position of some housing with care schemes is unclear. Whether or not such schemes are required to register as a care home may depend not only on whether or not residents have a tenancy and 'their own front door', but also on whether they can make a free choice on moving to this type of accommodation, even if another company provides the care (see Clements, 2004, p 162). Because of the difference in funding arrangements, tenants in sheltered accommodation have a higher disposable income than those in residential care; the former are funded through Housing Benefit in addition to receiving full pension entitlement; the latter are means tested on all their income, retaining only a small personal allowance.

Consideration, however, should also be given to the circumstances in which a tenancy in sheltered accommodation can be terminated. There may be a provision in the lease enabling the landlord to seek possession if the resident becomes too frail to manage. Differences of perception about the stage at which this is reached can be adjudicated in court, as a termination cannot be enforced without a possession order. The Disability Discrimination Act 1995 may protect people with a disability from less favourable treatment, at least if they do not cause harm to the health and safety of their neighbours. This applies also to people with mental health problems whose behaviour is attributable to their illness (*North Devon Homes v Brazier* [2003] EWHC 574). In addition, ss 13 and 16 of the Disability Discrimination Act 2005 make it unlawful for landlords to discriminate without justification against a person with disabilities or to fail to take reasonable steps to provide an auxiliary aid or service to facilitate their enjoyment of the tenancy. The landlord must show that any refusal of consent to proposed improvements to the premises by the tenant was reasonable (Cafferkey, 2005).

Supporting People

The Supporting People programme (www.spkweb.org.uk) is a recent innovation to help vulnerable people requiring limited support in the community to receive assistance from local authorities, often in combination with health care providers, the Probation Service and local voluntary agencies. Supporting People replaces some of the financial support for services previously provided under the Housing Benefit regime. Services must be housing related and provided as part of an agreed package of support. People receiving Housing Benefit are exempt from charging, as are those receiving 'short-term' services (defined as for up to two years) to assist in independent living.

Homelessness

A substantial number of older people may have housing needs that bring them within the scope of the legislation on homelessness. Accommodation that has become unsuitable because of disability or disrepair, or family conflicts, may be precipitating factors. Part VII of the Housing Act 1996 requires four conditions to be satisfied before a local authority owes the 'full housing duty' to a person seeking assistance. They must:

- be homeless
- be in priority need
- not be homeless intentionally
- not have a local connection elsewhere.

The definition of homelessness is wider that that of rooflessness; people living in crisis accommodation, refuges and night shelters are homeless, as are those who have no accommodation that it is reasonable for them to occupy. A person who is threatened with homelessness will qualify if they are likely to become homeless within 28 days. Local authorities are required to provide advice and assistance to any people who are homeless, but it is only people in 'priority need' who are owed a duty by the local authority to ensure that accommodation becomes available for their occupation (s 193 of the Housing Act

1996). The category of priority need includes those who are vulnerable as a result of old age, mental illness or handicap, physical disability or other special reason. In considering vulnerability, authorities should have regard to medical advice and where appropriate seek social services' assistance. Entitlement to accommodation may, however, be lost because of a further finding that the applicant is homeless intentionally. It is also for the local authority to establish intentionality, not for the applicant to disprove it. In any case, people who are intentionally homeless will still have a right to temporary accommodation (usually for 28 days) to give them a reasonable opportunity of securing their own accommodation independently of the local authority.

Even if the above qualifying criteria are established, a local authority may refer a person who has no local connection with their own area, but who does have a local connection with the area of another authority. 'Local connection' is not to be confused with 'ordinary residence' under s 21 of the National Assistance Act 1948 (see page 16), but may also be established by family association or employment in another area. However, a person who is at risk of violence in that other area should not be referred on. If a person who is in priority need and not intentionally homeless has no local connection with the area of any other housing authority in Britain, then the duty to secure accommodation rests with the authority to which the application is made.

The Housing Act 1996 has been amended in some important respects by the Homelessness Act 2002, which has created a greater emphasis on inter-agency cooperation by the requirement to produce a local homelessness strategy. When faced with an adverse decision by housing authorities, reference should first be made to the *Code of guidance on homelessness* (DCLG, 2006). At the same time, social workers should be aware that their own agency may have residual duties towards homeless people as one aspect of their community care needs. For example, in *Batantu v Islington London Borough Council* [2000] All ER (D) 1744, a man with mental ill health and his family living in a high-rise block were held to be entitled to rehousing by the local authority following a community care assessment which clearly identified a housing need under s 21 of the National Assistance Act 1948. Similarly, in *Barrett v Enfield London Borough Council* [2001] 2 AC 550 (see page 48) a disabled mother of six children who was intentionally homeless was nevertheless owed a duty to provide suitable housing by her local authority following a finding that her Article 8 rights had been breached. Arguments on the basis of family support are likely therefore to be the most potent in challenging adverse decisions on homelessness. In terms of the provision of accommodation, however, local authorities may consider cost when deciding that it is not reasonably practicable to secure that accommodation is provided within their district; in *R (Calgin) v Enfield London Borough Council* [2005] EWHC 1716, it was seen as acceptable to place a family from Enfield in accommodation in Birmingham.

Entering residential care

Changes in the funding arrangements for residential care, with top-up funding being removed from the Department for Work and Pensions' budget to individual local authorities, were designed to ensure that no one entered residential care supported by public funding without the appropriateness of that move being assessed (McDonald, 2006). Section 21 of the National Assistance Act 1948 in general applies only to people aged 18 or over (s 21(1)(c)) who are ordinarily resident in the area of the local authority. 'Ordinary residence' is of central concern in defining the extent of the local authority's duty and is defined in LAC (93)7 (DH, 1993b) and by common law. Scarman J in *Shah v London Borough of Barnet* [1983] 2 AC 309 defined ordinary residence as "the voluntary adoption of a place of abode for settled purposes and with some degree of continuity". Some older people may be living away from their usual places of abode because they have been living with family or because they have been in hospital or another type of residential accommodation for a period of time. It is likely that people who have moved in with family in order to receive care will be considered to have relocated (*R v Waltham Forest London Borough Council ex parte Vale* (1985) *The Times*, 25 February). Other situations are covered by LAC (93)7, the effect of which is that:

- people placed in residential accommodation in another local authority's area generally retain their ordinary residence;
- self-funders who move to residential accommodation themselves without being 'placed' by the local authority usually become ordinarily resident in the new area;
- agreements for a move from long-stay hospitals to care accommodation in the community under joint funding arrangements under s 28A of the National Assistance Act 1948 should specify ordinary residence;
- other patients discharged from hospitals, prisons and other establishments will normally be deemed to be ordinarily resident

in the area in which they were ordinarily resident before being admitted to that establishment.

Disputes about ordinary residence between authorities are to be determined by the Secretary of State. Clements (2004) sees difficult questions of ordinary residence as likely to arise from the Community Care (Delayed Discharges) Act 2003, as responsibility for the assessment process and reimbursement liability depends on the NHS body serving notice upon the correct local authority.

Meaning of 'residential accommodation'

In the majority of cases, 'residential accommodation' under s 21 of the National Assistance Act 1948 will mean accommodation in a care home, but the definition is wide enough to include ordinary housing. As Hale LJ stated in *R (Wahid) v Tower Hamlets London Borough Council* [2002] EWCA Civ 287:

> It can no longer be assumed that a need for care and attention can only be properly met in an institutional setting. There are people who are undoubtedly in need of care and attention for whom local authority social services authorities wish to provide residential accommodation in ordinary housing.

In *R v Bristol City London Borough Council ex parte Penfold* [1998] 1 CCLR 315, the social services authority was held to owe a duty to assess a person who appeared to be in need of community care services because of a difficult social and psychiatric history, even though she was ineligible for housing under the homelessness legislation. So, it may be possible to argue that accommodation in ordinary housing, with support services, is still a lawful use of s 21 of the National Assistance Act 1948.

Need for care and attention

Section 21 also requires that the person should be "in need of care and attention not otherwise available to them" (s 21(1)(c)). The responsibility of the National Asylum Support Service (NASS) is limited to asylum seekers who are "destitute or likely to become destitute" (s 95). This means that local authorities continue to have a duty to provide accommodation under s 21 of the National Assistance

Act 1948 to those who have a need of accommodation because of disability or old age (*R (on the application of Westminster City Council) v NASS* [2002] 1 WLR 2956). This means that older asylum seekers may retain the support of local communities rather than be subject to dispersal in the way in which younger people will be.

What is the effect of being able to pay for one's care on the local authorities' duty under s 21? Generally speaking, it will mean that the placement is not in consequence of a duty under s 21 and is not therefore publicly funded. This is advantageous to self-funders because it means that they can claim Attendance Allowance (or Disability Living Allowance if under the age of 65) whereas those supported by the local authority cannot do so beyond the first 28 days of the placement (see page 129). The situation is problematic in two circumstances: when self-funders start to struggle to meet their fees as their capital diminishes and when older people or their families are left without advice or support to find accommodation on their own – a not uncommon situation.

The well-known *Sefton* judgment (*R v Sefton Metropolitan Borough Council ex parte Help the Aged* [1997] 4 All ER 532) concerned an attempt by Sefton Council to refuse financial support for any person already in residential accommodation until their capital fell below £1,500 (far below the capital limit contained in the Charging for Residential Accommodation Guidance at that time). The Court of Appeal declared that such a policy was unlawful, but the issue is now a matter of statute law since s 53 of the Health and Social Care Act 2001 has inserted a new subsection (2A) into s 21 of the National Assistance Act 1948, which says that for the purpose of deciding whether care and attention are 'otherwise available', a local authority shall disregard so much of the person's capital as does not exceed the capital limit under the current charging guidance. Policy guidance LAC (98)19 (DH, 1998b) clarifies the second situation by stating that even if a person may not need the local authority to provide care and attention for financial reasons, their involvement in placement may be required because the person lacks mental capacity or has no family or friends able to help. Arguably, the requirements of this guidance are not met simply by giving individuals or families a list of care homes locally and asking them to make their own arrangements.

Section 21 speaks of the 'need' for care and attention and it is here that the local authority eligibility criteria take effect. 'Need' will be interpreted in accordance with the principles of the *Gloucestershire* case (see page 23), which enables local authorities to take resources into account when determining what needs are eligible. However, such a decision must follow a proper assessment that focuses not only on physical needs, but also on psychological and social needs. A local authority will be acting unlawfully therefore if it restricts residential accommodation to those with physical frailty or a recognised mental disorder, or refuses to continue to support people who were previously self-funding in their accommodation solely on the basis of cost. Good practice would involve the provision of appropriate information about the range of accommodation on offer, with an opportunity to visit individual homes to compare their facilities and their philosophies of care (McDonald, 2006).

Older people who do not have family or friends nominated to speak for them may be in need of advocacy services. What has previously been good practice will now become a legal requirement. Section 39 of the Mental Capacity Act 2005 requires a mental capacity advocate to be appointed when a local authority is considering providing long-term accommodation either under the National Assistance Act 1948 or under s 117 of the Mental Health Act 1983. An advocate is to be appointed where the older person lacks capacity and the decision maker is satisfied that there is no person other than one engaged in providing care or treatment in a professional capacity or for remuneration whom it would be to appropriate to consult in determining what would be in the service user's best interests. The advocate has access to local authority and health records to assist them in this role.

Unfortunately, once having made the decision, waiting lists can be lengthy, and choice limited. Across all sectors in 2003 there were 74,000 fewer residential care beds than in 1996 (Laing and Buisson, 2003). The balance of care provision between sectors has fundamentally changed since 1993, with local authorities now minority providers of residential care for older people; in 2004, only 17% of publicly funded placements were made in the local authority sector (DH, 2005a). There is no legal obligation on local authorities within a mixed economy of care to continue to make their own direct provision (*R v Wandsworth London Borough Council, ex parte Beckwith* [1996] All ER 129).

Once the resource provision decision has been made that a person is eligible for residential care, a place has to be provided within a reasonable time. Holding people on a waiting list because of a shortage of resources is not uncommon; in *R v Lanarkshire County Council ex parte McGregor* [2000] 4 CCLR 188, the applicant was on a list of 199 people, but it was successfully argued that the local authority could not refuse to make provision for his needs. The use of an allocation panel as a prioritising device *after* the decision on eligibility had been made was unlawful because it was clearly a response to a funding crisis. If no places are available at the local authority's usual cost then it may need to purchase accommodation elsewhere to meet its duty to individuals (Clements, 2004).

Choice in accommodation

Choice in residential care is critical but it is also threatened by shortage of resources. Unfortunately, the National Assistance Act 1992 (Choice of Accommodation) Directions 1992 and Guidance (LAC (2004)20) (DH, 2004f) are rarely drawn to the attention of prospective residents or their families. The policy behind these directions is to prevent older people from being placed in accommodation without consideration of their choice of setting or location. Local authorities commonly have lists of approved providers, or may adopt policies asking social workers, for example, to give priority to filling vacant places in local authority accommodation, in preference to other choices. The 1992 directions should act as a safeguard against the misuse of this discretion. They state that if a person (or their carer if that person is unable to express a preference) expresses a preference for particular accommodation (known as 'preferred accommodation') within the UK the authority must arrange for care in that accommodation provided that:

- the preferred accommodation appears to the authority to be suitable in relation to his or her needs as assessed by the authority;
- the cost of making arrangements would not require the authority to pay more than it would usually expect to pay having regard to the assessed needs;
- the preferred accommodation is available;
- the person in charge of the accommodation will provide it subject to the authority's usual terms and conditions.

Clements (2004, p 166) cites a decision of the local government ombudsman (Complaint 97/A/3218 against Merton London Borough Council) as authority for saying that a local authority will be guilty of maladministration if it fails to explain clearly to clients and their carers what their rights are under the directions, or if it puts the onus on them to find accommodation at an acceptable cost to the authority. In other words, individuals should not bear the consequences of deficiencies in the market for residential care in their area.

The scope of the directions was tested in *R v Avon County Council, ex parte M* [1994] 2 FCR 259. Mark Hazell was a young man with

Down's syndrome living in Avon who challenged through the complaints procedure, and later by judicial review, his authority's failure to find a placement for him at the Home Farm Trust. Expert evidence was called to show that Mark's desire for certainty over his placement had become a psychological need. Placement at the Home Farm Trust was thus not only preferred accommodation; it was the only placement that could meet his needs. In the case of older people, it may similarly be the case that only a familiar or local placement can properly meet their needs.

Issues of 'preferred' accommodation should be resolved before approaches are made to relatives to 'top up' the difference between the actual cost of the accommodation and the local authority's contribution. Often in practice, a direct approach is made to relatives in every case where accommodation is over the usual limit; this is misleading. The directions say only that the local authority is required to *accept* (not ask for) a third party to 'top up', subject to the local authority being satisfied as to the ability of the third party to maintain payments. Here caution is advised, for increases in the cost of care may not fall equally on the local authority and the person topping up. The resident is not able personally to top up fees except where they have entered into a deferred payment scheme with the local authority under the provisions of s 53 of the Health and Social Care Act 2001 (see page 133). It is worth noting that the right to preferred accommodation extends also to existing residents who wish to move to different accommodation. Also, a preference to move to another area of the country closer to family or friends may in itself be a psychological need, in which case the local authority of ordinary residence will be expected to pay the current rate for accommodation in that other area, even though it may be a more expensive part of the country. Patients in NHS-funded care do not have a statutory right of choice, although their wishes may be taken into account. Avoidance of delayed discharges may lead to interim placements in care homes being made pending the preferred accommodation becoming available, but it is clear (DH, 2003c) that such placements must still be able to meet the assessed care needs of the patient.

Contractual issues

Local authorities will contract with homes in the independent sector to provide care, and usually carry lists of 'approved providers'. There are clear links between the quality and the cost of care. Private providers, however, have no 'right' to be considered for such a list, and local authorities can give preference to their own in-house service (*R v Cumbria County Council ex parte Cumbria Professional Care Ltd* [2000] 3 CCLR 79). On the other hand, local authorities may impose more stringent contractual requirements on private sector homes than national minimum standards require. Where local authorities make placements under s 21 of the National Assistance Act 1948 they are responsible for payment in full, recovering charges from the resident according only to their assessed needs. However, under s 26(3A) of the National Assistance Act 1948 it is possible by agreement for the resident to enter into a contractual relationship to pay the assessed charge direct to the care home. The NHS is also responsible for providing continence services and supplies to nursing home residents, not the local authority or the resident.

Residents who are self-funding have to sign increasingly complex contracts, but few consult lawyers before signing (Bielanska, 2004). The Office of Fair Trading (2003) has published *A guide on unfair contract terms in care home contracts*. Terms that are likely to be unfair are: a liability to pay fees for termination of the contract beyond a four-week period; an unlimited right to sell possessions to meet unpaid fees; and exclusion of liability for negligence. Under s 2 of the Unfair Contract Terms Act 1977, terms that seek to exclude liability for death or personal injury caused by negligence are always void (Bielanska, 2004).

Closure of care homes

The closure of residential resources in both the independent and statutory sectors has led to discussion of the applicability of the Human Rights Act 1998 to residential care. In the *Coughlan* case (see page 60) it was accepted by the Court of Appeal that the health authority could break its promise of a home for life in that long-stay setting only if an overriding public interest required it, thus prioritising residents' rights to private and family life under Article 8 of the European Convention. However, later cases showed the reluctance of the courts to accept that thresholds for intervention based on Article 8 or Article 2 (the right to life) or Article 3 (protection from cruel, inhuman or degrading treatment or punishment) had been met. So, in *R (Dudley and Whitbread and others) v East Sussex County Council* [2003] EWHC 1093 Admin, Maurice Kay J considered that the local authority had justification under Article 8 for closing a residential home for older people on the basis of limited financial resources and demographic pressures created by a greater number of over-65s compared to any other local authority.

Nor did the evidence point to a breach of Article 2 in showing that the life of any particular resident was at risk. Additionally, in a review of the status of HSC 1998/048 (DH, 1998c), the individual risk assessments that the guidance required in transfers from NHS settings were held not to be something to which the local authority had to have regard. It seems therefore that strategic considerations on the deployment of resources are likely to be given precedence over individual claims based on Human Rights Act principles unless there is clear evidence of serious, and probably deliberate, harm.

The most limiting judgment in the field of human rights law and its application to residential care is the judgment of the Court of Appeal in *R (Heather, and others) v The Leonard Cheshire Foundation and the Attorney General* [2002] All ER 936. In that case it was decided that the Foundation was not a public body, and therefore not subject to the requirements of the Human Rights Act because it had no statutory powers, even though it accepted residents funded by the local authority. Although the judgment is subject to appeal, the failure to protect individual interests within the commissioning processes of agencies, led Age Concern to raise doubts about structural issues in the protection given to older people:

> An interpretation of the Act which results in older people having little protection against infringement of their civil rights by private individuals and organisations raises issues about the contracting out of statutory services which have a profound effect on people's welfare – such as health and social services – to the independent sector. (Age Concern, 2004)

Protection of human rights therefore remains the responsibility of the local authority through the imposition of contractual terms (ODPM, 2005). Paradoxically, given the development of supported living schemes, the decision of the Court of Appeal in the *Alternative Futures* case, *R (Moore) v Care Standards Tribunal* [2005] 1 WLR 2979, that some schemes remained legally 'care homes' has meant that deregistration has had limited impact. The registration regime is therefore hanging on to a protective role perhaps partly to fill the void left by the non-application of European Convention rights.

Regulation of residential care

From 1993, s 42(2) of the NHS and Community Care Act 1990 enabled local authorities to make placements in the voluntary or private sectors, so long as the accommodation was 'registered' under the Registered Homes Act 1984. The Care Standards Act 2000 extended registration and inspection to local authority services as well as those in the independent sector; it also set up an independent body, the National Care Standards Commission (NCSC), as the responsible registration and inspection authority for all types of care homes, including care homes with nursing. In April 2004, the NCSC was superseded by the Commission for Social Care Inspection (CSCI) as a result of the enactment of s 102 of the Health and Social Care (Community Health and Standards) Act 2003. There is now parity between the different sectors of care, and greater uniformity of standards, now that regulation is focused on one national body, albeit operating at a regional level.

Advising proprietors of residential care homes and their residents which conditions of registration are legally enforceable and which are simply advisory has always been a complex business (McDonald and Taylor, 1995). The Care Standards Act 2000, like the Registered Homes Act before it, raises difficult definitional issues about eligibility for registration, and contains both civil and criminal sanctions for its breach. The Act is also supported by regulations, guidance and 'national minimum standards', which together create a complex regime, elements of which have legal authority, and elements of which are merely persuasive, and 'good practice'.

It is useful to bear in mind throughout, Ridout's (2003) assessment of reasons why registration and inspection regimes are needed in an area of mixed public and commercial provision which deals with vulnerable people:

> Regulation arises out of a perceived need to control the activities of persons in their dealings with others, so as to protect those others and to ensure that society as a whole is satisfied that those in need of such protection are protected and are seen to be protected. (Ridout, 2003, p 7)

At the same time, any regulatory regime that operates in a scarce market has to draw a balance between 'policing' and 'supporting' good enough practice (CSCI, 2006). The registration and inspection of residential care faces problems common to all regulatory systems:

policing versus consultancy; rules versus discretion; stringency versus accommodation (Day et al, 1996), which render the pursuit of 'national standards' complex and illusory.

Definition of 'registered care home'

Section 3 of the Care Standards Act 2000 defines a 'care home' as follows:

> For the purposes of this Act, an establishment is a care home if it provides accommodation, together with nursing or personal care, for any of the following persons ... −
>
> persons who are or have been ill;
> persons who have or who have had a mental disorder [under s 121(1) mental disorder means 'mental illness, arrested or incomplete development of mind, psychopathic disorder, and any other disorder or disability of mind'];
> persons who are disabled or infirm;
> persons who are or have been dependent on alcohol or drugs.

Under the Registered Homes Act 1984 'board' was required in addition to personal care, but this is no longer the case, thus making registrable establishments where people prepare and cook their own food. 'Personal care' is not defined; it is likely to be interpreted more widely than "assistance with bodily functions" (s 121(9)), and to include emotional and psychological as well as physical care (Clements, 2004). The fact that care and accommodation are provided by separate organisations (as with many housing with care schemes) is not conclusive that the establishment is not registrable as a care home.

If the accommodation of people requiring nursing is authorised, the care home can be described as a 'care home with nursing', the category that replaces 'nursing home' registration. All care homes are registrable, the former category of 'small homes' having been abolished.

Range of people who are required to register under the Act

It is a criminal offence for a person to carry on or manage a care home without being registered (s 1 of the Care Standards Act 2000).

Both the proprietor or 'registered provider' and the manager of the care home must be registered. Personal accountability is emphasised by requiring a corporate body to give the name of an individual who is responsible for supervising the management of the care home, although there is no legal limit on the number of establishments in respect of which an individual can be nominated. The 'manager' of a care home must be an individual and will be responsible for the day-to-day running of the establishment in accordance with registration requirements. This may not be their only source of accountability, as Ridout (2003, p 58) makes clear:

> A care home manager who holds professional responsibilities will owe duties in respect of conduct of management and discharge of duties at a professional level to the relevant professional body ... as well as to the business owner under the appointment or contract of employment.

Both the registered provider and manager must be 'fit' to carry on the running of the home, and will be required to attend a 'fit person' interview, as well as to provide medical certificates, bank references and criminal record certificates. A fee is payable for registration and generally registration is not transferable.

Conditions of registration

Section 5(3) of the Registered Homes Act 1984 limited conditions to those relating to the numbers, ages, sex and category of people to be registered. Section 13(3) of the Care Standards Act 2000 says that an application may be granted either unconditionally or subject to such conditions as the registration authority sees fit. This is a very wide discretion, particularly as breaching conditions of registration "without reasonable excuse" is an offence (s 24). Applicants will be refused if they cannot show that they are able to comply with conditions of registration, and final approval may not be given until the home is built, furnished, commissioned and staffed (Ridout, 2003).

Regulations and national minimum standards

Proprietors and managers of registered care homes are of course subject to the general law as well as the law specific to care standards. This would include legislation on health and safety at work, and the Medicines Act 1968, and, where appropriate, the protective provisions of the Mental Health Act 1983. Much of the detail of the Care Standards Act 2000 is contained in regulations. The Care Homes Regulations 2001 are mandatory and relate to 'premises', 'accommodation' and 'facilities' (DH, 2003e). The premises must be fit to be used, suitable for their purpose and located in an area appropriate to meet the needs of the service users. Accommodation must be 'adequate' for both individual and communal needs; facilities such as bathrooms and lavatories must also be 'sufficient'; and facilities for meeting visitors must be 'suitable'. Obviously these are very broad requirements; for example, reg 23 of the Care Homes Regulations on the physical design and layout of premises says only that the size and layout of rooms used by service users must be suitable for their needs. What this means in practice for older people is described in the minimum standards for care homes for older people (DH, 2003e), one of a number of standards documents produced as guidance by the Secretary of State under the new powers given by s 23 of the Care Standards Act 2000. Such national minimum standards are an attempt to standardise practice in decision making and must be 'taken into account' by the CSCI when considering registration and the imposition of conditions for registration, variation of any conditions and enforcement of compliance with the Act and regulations. They are not, however, legally binding.

The minimum standards for care homes for older people were reviewed in 2003 (DH, 2003e); for homes that had been subject to registration before April 2002, a transitional period was allowed to enable changes to be made to the structure and fabric of the premises. However, the standards were intended to become immediately applicable to all new registrations. The reaction was the closure of homes that could not meet the new standards and a revision of the standards together with a statement that they would only be applied to entirely new provisions, not to care homes that had previously been exempt from registration, including local authority homes. However, this relaxation did not mean that owners did not have to meet the requirements of the Care Standards Act or the regulations, simply that the interpretation of the regulations was to be less rigidly applied.

An important innovation of the Care Standards Act is the requirement (Care Homes Regulations 2001, reg 4) that every home should have a 'statement of purpose' to serve as a standard by which the operation of the home can be judged for the purpose of registration and inspection. The statement of purpose must describe all the facilities and services that the home provides, such as care arrangements, food preparation, social activities and hygiene. In addition, the process of care planning is facilitated by the requirement that there should be an individual assessment of need for each prospective resident (reg 14), and a service user plan for each resident (reg 15). Schedule 1 of the Care Home Regulations requires the home to specify in its statement of purpose the qualifications and experience of the registered provider and registered manager, and the number, qualifications and experience of the staff working at the home and how staff may refer complaints. A registered care home with nursing, for example, must have a qualified nurse permanently on duty and all homes are required to provide training for staff who will be handling medicines.

Sanctions and appeals

The previous requirement of two inspections a year by the CSCI has been replaced by a minimum of one inspection every three years (CSCI (Fees and Frequency of Inspection) (Amendment) Regulations 2006, SI 2006/517). This enables the CSCI to focus on services that have a greater need to improve; 'themed' visits will also focus on national and local issues, with a greater emphasis throughout on people using the services (CSCI, 2006). The regulations relate also to domiciliary care providers and nursing agencies. Reports arising from inspections are public documents. There is a power to interview in private any manager, member of staff or resident. It is a criminal offence to obstruct or without reasonable cause to fail to comply with the requirements of an inspection. Power to effect the cancellation of registration is contained in s 14 of the Care Standards Act 2000 for conviction for offences under the Act, or for breach of the conditions of registration, for false statement on a registration application, non-payment of the annual registration fee or lack of financial viability. This procedure may also be used to vary or remove existing conditions, or impose new conditions. There is a procedure under s 20 for the urgent cancellation of registration by application to a magistrates' court where there is a serious risk to life, health or well-being. One difficulty is that neither the CSCI nor the local authority has the power, without the consent of the owners, to carry on the business on their behalf, although the local authority will have a duty under s 21 of the National Assistance Act 1948 to provide accommodation. Appeal against refusal or cancellation of registration or variation of a condition of registration lies to the Care Standards Tribunal.

Case study 3: Housing disputes

Helen Hall is 80 years old. She lives in a sheltered housing complex that is privately owned. Other residents have made frequent complaints about noise at night and about Helen's hoarding of rubbish in the flat that they claim is a health hazard. The on-site manager has tried to tackle Helen about these issues but Helen has said that there is no problem – the neighbours just don't understand her way of life is different from theirs and that it is they who are harassing her.

What are the legal issues and how might the situation be resolved?

Further reading

Ridout, P. (2003) *Care standards: A practical guide*, Bristol: Jordans.
Describes the process of registering and inspecting care homes for older people and the standards that are to be applied.

Oldman, C. (2000) *Blurring the boundaries: A fresh look at housing and care provision for older people*, Brighton: Pavilion.
Research-based findings of the potential of housing with care schemes for older people, compared with traditional models of residential care.

Arden, A. and Hunter, C. (2003) *Manual of housing law* (7th edn), London: Thompson, Sweet and Maxwell.
A comprehensive manual of housing law for specialist practitioners, but clearly written and accessible to non-lawyers.

FOUR

Financial management

For most of our lives we retain personal control over our own financial and business affairs, signing our own cheques and making our own decisions, however eccentric they may seem to the outside world. If health begins to fail as we get older the management of such matters can become an increasing burden, often spiralling out of control before the magnitude of the problem has been appreciated. Social workers find dealing with financial matters particularly complex, involving as they do both practical and ethical issues, often requiring liaison with other professionals or organisations, and being sensitive to family expectations (Bradley and Manthorpe, 1995).

There are three ways in which at least an element of dealing with such matters can be handed over to a third party.

- appointeeship
- power of attorney
- Court of Protection – receivership

The first two involve choice on the part of the person whose affairs are concerned. However, if understanding has generally been lost to such an extent that choice cannot be exercised, then the third option will apply and the court will make most decisions. The vital points to remember are that the older person must trust their agent, and the agent must bear in mind that they are handling someone else's money and are accountable to them for its management. Also, any control given over is in relation to business and financial affairs, not the physical person of the individual concerned.

There are different medico/legal tests of capacity depending on the particular transactions or decisions which an individual is taking. For a definitive explanation of the various tests see *Assessment of mental capacity*, a joint publication of the British Medical Association and Law Society (2004).

Appointeeship

This is a system used by the Department for Work and Pensions whereby National Insurance Retirement Pension and other benefits (for example, Attendance Allowance, Pension Credit) are paid on behalf of the claimant to an agreed third party (the appointee). The Department prefers a relative, although it will pay to a friend or professional adviser. It does not like to pay direct to the proprietors of residential or nursing homes, and local authorities tend not to allow their employees (for example, home carers, wardens of sheltered accommodation) to be named. The claimant has to agree to the third party being appointed, as does the Department, which sends one of its officers to interview both parties, in particular checking on the suitability of the third party to be collecting someone else's benefits. The appointment is indefinite until given up by the appointee or revoked by the claimant or the Department. The appointee undertakes to the Department to pay back overpaid benefits which they receive on the claimant's behalf, and to notify the Department of relevant changes in circumstance. The Department has encouraged individuals to have their benefits paid into a nominated bank account (preferably in their own name), but it is still possible for an appointee to collect the benefits, weekly, from a Post Office, using the newly introduced card system.

Power of attorney

This is a document that appoints another or others (the attorney) to act in connection with the business and financial affairs of the donor. It is vital that, whatever type of power of attorney is selected, the donor has sufficient mental understanding at the time the power is signed to comprehend the nature of the document and its implications. Currently powers of attorney can only deal with business and financial affairs and not health care decisions – there is power over the purse not the person – but the introduction of lasting powers of attorney under the Mental Capacity Act 2005, due to be available from April 2007, will also allow for an attorney to make health care decisions if specified within the lasting power.

If the donor wishes to appoint the attorney for a 'one-off' transaction, such as to sell a property, the short form, 'ordinary' power of attorney, as defined by s 10 of the Powers of Attorney Act 1971, should be sufficient. This type of document fails and the attorney has no power and no legal protection once the transaction for which it is to be used has been completed or the donor's mental health has failed so that they no longer understand the actions which their attorney is taking.

If the donor is looking to appoint an attorney to handle everyday transactions indefinitely, be it now or in the future, then the newer 'enduring power of attorney', as created by the Enduring Powers of Attorney Act 1985, and subsequent statutory instruments, should be used until replaced by the lasting power of attorney under the Mental Capacity Act 2005. The document is in a set wording laid down by statutory instrument: the Court of Protection (Enduring Powers of Attorney) Rules 2001 (SI 2001/825). It is in three sections: an explanatory first part warning the donor of the implications of entering into the document; a middle part identifying the power of attorney as being that of a particular donor with personal details such as name and age and which the donor signs; and the third part being signed by the attorney where they acknowledge the responsibilities that they are taking on and their obligations under the law.

The donor can give 'general power' to their attorney so that it will operate in connection with all financial affairs, or put in any restrictions they like, not to sell a particular asset or that the attorney can only act under the power once the donor is no longer mentally capable of managing their own affairs.

For an enduring power of attorney to be valid it must be made while the donor still has mental capacity, but their level of understanding does not have to be such that they can actually manage their own affairs within the terms of s 94(2) of the Mental Health Act 1983.

The case of *Re K* [1988] 2 FLR 15 decided that the donor only needs to understand, at the time of signing the enduring power of attorney:

- that the attorney will be able to exert complete control over the donor's affairs (if such be the terms of the power);
- that the attorney will in general be able to do anything with the donor's property that they themselves could have done (if such be the terms of the power);
- that the authority will continue if the donor should be or become mentally incapable;
- that if the donor should become mentally incapable the power will be irrevocable without confirmation by the court.

In *Re K*-type situations, where the donor's mental capacity would appear to be starting to fail, the attorney may well have to look to registering the enduring power of attorney with the Public Guardianship Office almost immediately after it has been entered into.

While the donor has understanding, they direct their attorney's actions to pay this bill but not that. Once the attorney believes the donor is or is becoming mentally incapable of managing their affairs, then the attorney is legally obliged under the Act to register the enduring power of attorney in the Public Guardianship Office. As the donor no longer understands, they cannot control the attorney's actions and so authorise them. So as to continue to have the authority to handle the donor's affairs, the attorney has to have the protection of registration. The donor and at least three members of their family, as detailed by statute, have to be informed by notice of the application to register. This gives a chance for objections to be raised and the court to consider the validity of the proceedings. A one-off fee (currently £120) is payable although the court has the power to waive the fee, generally in cases where the donor's assets total less than local authority capital limits for paying for services. The attorney's authority is temporarily limited to doing those acts that are necessary to protect the donor's affairs only. If there are no objections or the court considers any objections raised to be invalid, the power is registered and the attorney can resume acting under the power as they did before. But now they reach the decisions and, if anything controversial arises, they can apply to the Court of Protection for guidance. An attorney should keep accounts as to how they are dealing with their donor's finances as it always open to the Public Guardianship Office to call for them. The attorney may also have to explain to their donor's executors, after the donor's death, how they have dealt with matters during the donor's lifetime.

If an attorney is believed to be mishandling the finances of their donor (in addition to any criminal proceedings that may be brought), if the donor still has capacity they can revoke the appointment. If the enduring power of attorney has been registered, then the behaviour of the attorney needs to be brought to the attention of the court, which will both impound the power, cancel the registration and, possibly, bring the donor's finances within the control of the court by the appointment of a receiver. As a power of attorney is a document created by deed, so it can be revoked by the donor by a simple deed of revocation. The only proviso on this relates to enduring powers of attorney, which, although capable of revocation while unregistered, cannot be revoked once registered in the court.

Enduring powers of attorney will be replaced by lasting powers of attorney under the Mental Capacity Act 2005. These documents are proposed to come into force in April 2007 but their exact format is still being agreed. Such powers of attorney will have to be registered with the Public Guardianship Office (due to be renamed as the Office of the Public Guardian) before they can be brought into use, and will enable the attorney to make not only financial decisions, but also decisions relating to health and personal care. Lasting powers of attorney can be used both before and after the donor loses capacity with outcomes subject to both the principles of the Act and the donor's best interests. The principles include:

- the presumption that the donor has capacity to make their own decisions unless it is proved otherwise;
- all practicable steps must be taken to help the donor make their own decisions or to permit and encourage the donor to participate as fully as possible in any decisions affecting them;
- an unwise decision must not automatically be assumed to indicate a lack of capacity;
- anything done for or on behalf of the donor must be in their best interests;
- anything done for or on behalf of the donor should be the least restrictive of their basic rights and freedoms.

Existing enduring powers of attorney will continue to be valid after lasting powers of attorney come in, but no new enduring powers of attorney will be able to be made.

Court of Protection – receivership

If no valid enduring power of attorney has been signed and an individual is unable to manage their affairs because of mental incapacity, then, in order for such matters to be handled properly, there is no option but to apply to the Court of Protection. The court's authority is found in ss 93–113 of the Mental Health Act 1983. The court may sometimes insist on receivership, even if there is an enduring power of attorney, if it considers it is in the patient's interests to bring their affairs under the court's jurisdiction.

The court requires medical evidence (usually from the GP or a psychogeriatrician and for which they will charge a fee) on a standard form, that the individual (known as the patient) is mentally incapable so that the court has jurisdiction. The burden of proof rests on those asserting incapacity. In *Masterman-Lister v Brutton and Co; Masterman-Lister v Jewell and another* [2003] 3 All ER 162, the Court of Appeal held that the fact that the claimant had received severe head injuries in a road accident did not mean that he was presumed to continue to be incapacitated, without medical evidence being produced to satisfy the court. The court may, however, act retrospectively if there was good faith and no manifest disadvantage to the patient. It is worth checking with medical attendants first that any confusion arises from failing mental health (for example, Alzheimer's Disease) and not from alcohol abuse, adverse reaction to medication or an acute infection which, once diagnosed, can be controlled.

As well as medical evidence, the court requires a brief factual history of the patient, details of their assets and proposals as to what orders are sought. If there is only a small investment to which access is required, the court will issue a short form order authorising the release of the funds required. Where the individual runs their own home, or if there are several assets, and pensions to collect, the court needs to make more comprehensive provision for the handling of their affairs. This is done by way of a First General Order, which usually appoints a receiver, a named person, generally a relative, who is authorised to collect all future pensions and income from investments. The First General Order may go on to authorise the rationalisation of assets by the closure of small investments, the disposal of personal chattels and the sale of property and to specify the whereabouts of securities and valuables for safekeeping.

The receiver will have to be fidelity bonded, taking out an insurance against misappropriation of monies, the annual premium in respect of which is paid out of the patient's assets. The receiver will be expected to open a receivership bank account in their own name 'as receiver for the patient' and is encouraged to have all monies passing through this account. Generally, the court will require an annual account to be prepared, coinciding with the anniversary of the First General Order, and it is much easier to prepare the account if all transactions have gone through the bank. This is also a convenient time to suggest to the court any changes in policy, reinvestment etc. The receiver cannot touch capital unless specifically ordered to. If income is insufficient to meet residential home fees, then an approach is made to the court for a short order authorising the release of funds from a specific investment of the patient's.

In recent months the Court of Protection has introduced Empowerment Orders whereby professional receivers such as solicitors are appointed with more general power than that granted to lay receivers. In such cases the receiver can make decisions about access to capital or other investments without having to go back to the court for a further order.

The appointment of receivers will be replaced under the Mental Capacity Act 2005 by the appointment of deputies through a newly constituted Court of Protection. The court will have power to make 'one-off' orders to settle single questions but also to appoint a deputy to make ongoing decisions if there is no lasting power of attorney in place. In deciding what type of order to make the court must apply the Act's principles and 'best interests' checklist.

Where assets are jointly owned, such as bank accounts requiring joint signatures, or the matrimonial home, there can be problems if one of the parties is not capable of comprehending any transaction so that their signature is worthless. The court has the power to authorise someone else to sign, generally not the capable spouse as there are elements of trust law to be considered, so another, third person is involved to complete the transaction.

The court has power to make a statutory will on behalf of the patient if they no longer have testamentary capacity and have either no will or one sufficiently out of date to require alteration. Having considered evidence of the relatives, assets and the patient's likely views if they could express them, the court may order the making of a will on the patient's behalf.

There are many misunderstandings about the involvement of the Court of Protection. While the court is based in London (although this is due to change under the Mental Capacity Act 2005), it is dealt with by post and telephone, and physical appearance in the court building is rare – generally only if issues are being contested or a will or similar major matter is being considered. Appointments of receivers, selling properties and agreeing accounts are postal matters. The court procedure is generally slow and expensive, with varying fees being paid at different times depending on the transaction. If there is an emergency, the court staff and the Master will do their best to produce an order quickly. In addition to the court fees along the way, there is an annual percentage fee to the court, and legal fees for the work done. All of these come from the patient's assets. Despite this, the affairs have to be properly handled, and it gives everyone peace of mind to know things are being done correctly. Also, if tackled early enough, the proceedings often bring to light the fact that full benefits and tax allowances are not being claimed and that monies can be invested for a better return, so that the increased income generated will often make up for the costs necessarily expended.

One golden rule is to approach doctors, social workers and solicitors who are experienced in this type of work and not to be put off by bank and building society staff who do not understand the paperwork with which they will be presented as it will appear unusual. A response to this concern has, however, come from the British Bankers' Association (BBA, 2005), which has produced a leaflet of guidance on banking for mentally incapacitated customers (available at www.bba.org.uk).

Lifetime gifts

In anticipation of moving into permanent care, many people consider giving away the majority of their assets. Before committing themselves to such an irrevocable step, all the implications need to be considered carefully.

By giving away inheritance early, a parent may be giving up the only remaining form of control they have. Once the family have the monies or assets, they may no longer be so willing to visit or fulfil any other obligations. Once a gift is made, it cannot be recalled and, by its nature, no conditions can be imposed. From an Inheritance Tax 'death duty' point of view, such gifts may be ineffective. If, for example, an elderly parent transfers their house into the name of their child but continues to reside in the property, the gift is not tax effective, and will only become so once the parent moves out on a permanent basis. The following should also be considered:

- there may be Capital Gains Tax consequences on disposing of an asset during lifetime that would not arise if the asset passes on death;
- the gift might be considered as a deliberate deprivation of assets that will make the donor of the gift ineligible for means-tested benefits and may mean they will still be expected to pay for community care charges based on the assumption that the value of the asset remains within their estate;
- there may also be unforeseen consequences within the family should the beneficiary of the gift predecease the donor, become bankrupt or divorce.

Equity release schemes

Many older couples are asset rich but cash poor, with all value being tied up in the ownership of their home. Increasingly, they are taking advantage of equity release schemes whereby money is borrowed against the security of the property.

Generally the owner has to be at least 70 years old, or if a couple, have a combined age of 140 before they will be considered for such a scheme. The property is valued and the 'lender' then provides cash in return for a share of the property or a mortgage where the interest is rolled up and capital and accumulated interest repaid when the property is sold (generally on the move into a care home or death).

Care has to be taken with such schemes as the cash lump sum can mean a loss of means-tested benefits (such as Council Tax Benefit or Pension Credit) and the rolled-up interest can build into a considerable debt.

Undue influence

In recent years the courts have started to look much more closely into the relationship between the donor of any gifts or terms of a testator's will and the beneficiary of those gifts. If both parties have not taken independent advice as to all the consequences of their actions then it is quite likely that the gifts or the will may be set aside.

Most employers of carers have it as a term of their employment contract that an employee cannot accept gifts from one of their clients, either in their lifetime, or by will, subject to a de minimis rule, whereby they are allowed to receive a small token of appreciation, such as a box of chocolates. The provision does not protect donors from their relatives, their neighbours or privately arranged carers.

Unless what has happened can be clearly seen as the donor's intention then there is the possibility that things can be set aside due to 'undue influence' on the donor by the beneficiary or a related party. As everyone is subject to influence of varying types, the influence has to be proved to be 'undue', effectively coercion.

In *Aldridge and Hunt v Turner* [2004] EWHC 2768 (Ch) gifts of individually modest amounts were set aside because of their total value when added together. During his lifetime the deceased had given his son 62 separate sums which totalled £25,000. His regular income was less than £2,000 per month. While some of the transactions were legitimate, others were wholly unauthorised or deemed to have been made as a result of undue influence. The son was ordered to account back to the estate for the non-legitimate amounts.

In *Hammond v Osborn and another* [2002] EWCA Civ 885 an elderly bachelor living alone was befriended by a neighbour. As he became frailer the neighbour became more responsible for his care. Initially, using a legitimately obtained bank mandate, she accessed his funds for food and clothing. It was claimed on several occasions he wanted to give her some of his savings but that those requests were initially ignored. He was admitted to hospital and told her where he kept the paperwork relating to his investments and that he wanted to give them to her. With the help of her bank official son, the investments, worth over £297,000, were released and the monies transferred to her account. The elderly gentleman died shortly thereafter. The beneficiaries of his estate sought the return of the money and the Court of Appeal agreed. It was felt that the fact that Mrs Osborn had not encouraged the gifts was not enough. Independent advice should have been given particularly bearing in mind the fact that the assets gifted were worth approximately 90% of the value of the entire estate, so little was left for the donor to live on; he had not been informed of the value of the investments he was gifting; their realisation gave rise to a substantial tax liability; and, even if there was to be a reward to Mrs Osborn for her kindness, the amount of the gift was "wholly out of proportion to the kindness shown to him".

Employment rights in older age

Employment rights for older people in the UK have only recently been secured. The scope of anti-discriminatory legislation has been extended by the requirement of compliance with the EU's Employment Directive 2000/78/EC on Equal Treatment. The EU Directive requires member states to introduce legislation to prohibit both direct and indirect discrimination on the basis of disability, sexual orientation, religion and beliefs and also age. In respect of age, the requirement extends only to employment and vocational training. However, the experience of other countries has shown that legislation is not the only factor affecting employment levels of older people; change in attitude and flexible employment practices are also required. Some employers view the employment of older people positively in terms of reflecting the age profile of the local population. Examples of good practice, including part-time and seasonal working, are available at www.agepositive.gov.uk

Regulations in force from October 2006 are the Employment Equality (Age) Regulations 2006 (SI 2006/1031). Discrimination against older people may be either direct (less favourable treatment) or indirect (policies and practices that in fact discriminate against workers of a particular age). Both are subject to an objective justification test that might include efficiency, or providing promotion opportunities to retain key staff. An employer can never justify harassment and victimisation. There are exemptions from the law relating to length of service benefits, such as additional holiday, and 'genuine occupational requirements'. Employers are allowed positively to discriminate on the basis of age to encourage people to take up employment opportunities or access training, although actual selection based on age is not lawful. Nor is it unlawful to refuse to employ someone who is over the age of 65, the statutory 'default' retirement age.

Compulsory retirement under the age of 65, for both men and women, will be unlawful unless it can be justified. The employer must give six months' notice of retirement, but will have a duty to consider (not necessarily grant) a request by an employee to continue working. A claim of unfair dismissal by a person over 65 can only be based on the correct procedure not having been followed; for example an older person may wish to argue that the real reason for the employer's refusal to let them stay on at work over the agoe of 65 is that redundancies, although not imminent, are in the offing. The dismissal will still be fair if correct procedure has been followed, and the employer does not have to give reasons for their refusal. Thus it can be seen that the protection given by the 2006 regulations is only partial and does not amount to the removal of barriers to employment for older people.

The existence of multiple sources of discrimination, where age combines with disability or racial discrimination, may mean that complex legal arguments can be raised. Issues of human rights may also fall for consideration. Although the substantive law will not change, arguments relating to breaches of human rights and of anti-discriminatory legislation relating to race, gender, age and disability will in future come together under the jurisdiction of a single Commission for Equality and Human Rights. The Commission, which was created by the Equality Act 2006, will begin work in April 2007. The Commission will have positive duties to promote equality and to combat discrimination, and will also be able to support group actions to clarify and to enforce the law.

Pensions

State pensions

Age Concern has an excellent fact sheet (2006b) on state pensions. It explains the contribution conditions, including home responsibility protection, implications of deferring pensions and the effect of marriage and divorce on pensions. The amount of pension received depends on the number of national insurance contributions paid; it consists of a basic state pension plus an additional state pension (after April 1978) or Graduated Retirement Benefit based on contributions between April 1961 and April 1978. Pensions are not awarded automatically and have to be claimed. State pension is taxable and taken into account for entitlement to other means-tested benefits. It is possible currently to contract out of the additional state pension into occupational, personal or stakeholder pensions. Self-employed people do not have access to the additional state pension and may wish to make other arrangements (West, 2006). In 2010, pensionable age will be equalised at 65 for men and women. Despite the coming into force of the Civil Partnership Act (2004) in 2005, married women's pension rules will not apply to men in civil partnerships until this time. The European Court of Justice in the case of *Richards v Secretary of State for Works and Pensions (Case C-423/04)* (2006) has, however, held that the refusal to grant a pension to a male-to-female transsexual at the age of 60 was contrary to the European Economic Community (EEC) Directive 79/7 on equal treatment in social security matters. Men who are in receipt of Jobseeker's Allowance at the age of 60 can remain on benefit until 65, or they can move onto Pension Credit (see page 123). Age structures within society are thus clearly reflected in pension provision, with attendant assumptions of gender roles and withdrawal from employment.

Proposed changes

The Pensions White Paper (DWP, 2006a) proposes fundamental changes in the way in which pensions are calculated. The drivers are: a dependency ratio of people in employment compared to pensioners, currently at 27% but set to rise to 47% by 2050; and inequities in a system based on employment patterns in the 1940s. Briefly:

- it is proposed that the state pension age will rise incrementally to 68 by April 2046;
- for those retiring after 2010 only 30 years of national insurance contributions will be required to qualify for the full state pension (currently the requirement is 44 years for men and 39 for women);
- the link between pensions and earnings which was broken in 1980 will be restored probably from 2012, and will replace inflation-linked rises. There will be no catch-up payments for past years;
- a new basic National Pensions Saving Scheme for occupational pensions will begin in 2012; the funding will go into personal accounts that workers can take with them if they move jobs;

- from 2010 carers who spend 20 hours a week or more in caring will be able to accrue credits towards state pension;
- from 2012 the second state pension will become a flat rate benefit, regardless of national insurance contributions. Contracting out will be ended except for employers with final salary pension schemes that provide the equivalent of state benefits;
- the Financial Assistance Scheme that the government set up in 2004 partially to compensate victims of failed company pension schemes is to be extended to those who were then within 15 years of retirement, compared to within 3 years currently.

The emphasis is thus on a model of ageing which emphasises productivity in older age, flexibility in employment and the residual position of the welfare state.

Social security benefits

There is a wide range of social security benefits currently available to older people, both means tested and non-means tested. The Department for Work and Pensions that administers benefits is divided into a number of different agencies: the Pension Service, Jobcentre Plus (for those seeking employment) and the Disability and Carers Service. HM Revenue & Customs is the agency that administers Working Tax Credit and Child Tax Credit.

Being aware of the range and type of benefits available is a necessary part of effective working in community care; part of the assessor's role under the *Fair access to care services* (DH, 2002a) is maximising the income of service users to enable them to exercise choice, and to buy in resources not otherwise available. Getting all the benefits to which one is entitled can greatly improve an older person's quality of life (CSCI, 2005). The law in this area is, however, extremely complex, and the following is intended as a guide only; annual updates are published by, among others, Child Poverty Action Group and the Disability Alliance (see Appendix for contact details). Generally speaking, people of pensionable age will be moved from other benefits onto Pension Credit to avoid overlapping systems for claiming means-tested benefits and some benefits such as Disability Living Allowance have an upper age limit of 64 for a first claim.

Pension Credit

Pension Credit is a non-contributory benefit that may be classified as a top-up to retirement pension or other income. It has two parts: the guarantee credit that provides a basic income for single people or couples over 60; and a savings credit that is available to people over 65 who have savings below £6,000 (£10,000 if resident in a care home). Savings credit is intended to reward people who have a modest income additional to the state pension, say through an occupational pension. The maximum savings credit is £17.88 for a single person and £23.58 for a couple (2006 rates); this is based on qualifying income of £114.05 and £174.05, respectively (which is the level of the basic pension guarantee). There are, however, additions to the pension guarantee for people who are disabled or carers, or who own their own homes and have relevant housing costs. Basic pension guarantee is now unaffected by stays in hospital, however long.

Income Support

Although Pension Credit has replaced Income Support as a benefit for people of pensionable age, Income Support remains available to younger people not required to sign on for work or as a top-up to other benefits such as Severe Disablement Allowance, or income-based Jobseeker's Allowance. There are premiums for disability and for carers. Premiums for dependent children have now become Child Tax Credit, whether the recipient is in employment or not.

Social Fund

The Social Fund covers needs arising from exceptional circumstances that cannot be met from normal income. Eligibility is limited to those on means-tested benefits and includes those in receipt of Pension Credit. There are both discretionary and non-discretionary payments. For those aged 60 and over, savings of over £2,000 are taken into account (for younger people the threshold is £1,000).

Non-discretionary payments are maternity payments, payments for funeral expenses and cold weather payments. Funeral expenses for burial or cremation costs, travel and other expenses (up to a maximum of £700) are payable only to the person responsible for arranging the funeral, a test which has become narrower in recent years, and is usually limited to partners and close relatives. The person who died must have been resident in the UK, and costs are reclaimable from their estate. Cold weather payments, payable for periods of very cold weather, are paid automatically to eligible pensioners, people claiming disability benefits and households with children under the age of 5. They do not need to be claimed. The refusal of a non-discretionary payment may be subject of an appeal to a social security appeal tribunal.

Discretionary Social Fund payments are limited by local budgets set by the Department for Work and Pensions and are subject to internal review, not appeal. Although there is national guidance on priority groups (which includes older people) and district priorities (details of which should be publicly available), each case should be considered on its merits. Any person, not just those in receipt of benefits, can apply for a crisis loan for emergencies, being "the only way that serious damage or serious risk to health or safety can be prevented". Living expenses at the beginning of benefits claims may be paid by way of a crisis loan. Budgeting loans are available only to those continuously in receipt of eligible benefits for six months or more. The minimum loan is for £30, and they must normally be repaid in 78 weeks. Furniture, bedding, clothing and home repairs are a priority. Loans are not available for domestic assistance in the home, or for deposits to secure accommodation, as opposed to rent in advance. Community care grants (preferable to loans, when available, because they are non-repayable) are intended to cover: re-establishment in the community following a period in institutional or residential care; support to remain in the community; travel in the UK to cover domestic crisis or to visit a sick person; or a grant to move to more suitable accommodation. Usually a stay in residential care is relevant only if it is over three months or more in duration, but this is not an absolute rule. It is advisable to cost items sought, for example from a catalogue. Community care grants may also be claimed to allow a potential carer to move in with the person for whom they will provide care.

Other payments

Winter fuel payments are not means tested and are available to most people aged over 60 (even in work) who live in Britain. The payment for 2005/06 has been £200 per household, with an additional £100 if someone in the household is over the age of 80. Age eligibility is calculated from the week beginning the third Monday in September.

People over 60 who are in receipt of Pension Credit, income-based Jobseeker's Allowance, Housing Benefit or Council Tax Benefit may receive Warm Front grants to insulate their property to the value of £2,700. People over 60 in receipt of Attendance Allowance or Disability Living Allowance, but not on a means-tested benefit, may still be eligible for £1,500 worth of help. In addition to these benefits; television licences are free at the age of 75, and from April 2006, all local authorities are required to give free off-peak travel on public transport within their area to people aged 60 and over, as well as to those who have a disability.

Bereavement benefits

Bereavement benefits are payable only to people under pensionable age, both men and women, but depend upon the national insurance contributions of the spouse who has died. There is a lump sum bereavement payment of £2,000, a bereavement allowance paid to people aged 45 or over which is paid for 52 weeks and a Widowed Parent's Allowance for people with dependent children. People over pensionable age who are bereaved will receive a state pension from the outset; those on bereavement benefits who reach pensionable age will be moved onto Pension Credit, thus preventing an overlap of benefits. Although the Welfare Reform and Benefits Act 1999 introduced equal rights for widows and for widowers to state benefits in *R (Hooper) v Secretary of State for Work and Pensions* [2006] 1 All ER 487, the House of Lords, held that discrimination against men widowed before 2001 (when the Act came into force) was objectively justified. The reason given was on the grounds that widows were historically an economically disadvantaged class, and that therefore positive discrimination in their favour was justifiable. This means that men widowed before 2001 cannot retrospectively claim benefits to equalise their pension with that of women.

Incapacity Benefit

Incapacity Benefit has replaced Sickness Benefit and Invalidity Benefit for people below pensionable age who are unable to work due to sickness or disability and who have paid sufficient national insurance contributions. People who have been in employment move onto Incapacity Benefit after being in receipt of statutory sick pay for 26 weeks.

Eligibility for Incapacity Benefit is based on a personal capability assessment that satisfies one of two tests: the 'own occupation' test that applies for the first six months of incapacity; and the 'all work' test that applies thereafter, or from the beginning of a claim if there is no usual occupation. The assessment is based on a functional test of disability across a range of competences that cover both physical and mental impairments. Some people, for example those with early onset dementia or neurological disorders, will be deemed to have qualified for the benefit by virtue of the nature of their condition.

Changes to Incapacity Benefit are likely in the near future. The Green Paper on welfare reform (DWP, 2006b) proposes the replacement of Income Support and Incapacity Benefit with a single Employment and Support Allowance from 2008. This will include reform of the personal capability assessment to place a greater emphasis on functional capability for 'work-related activity'. It also proposes that people aged 50-59 will be required to take part in the 'New Deal' for retraining, and return to work. The emphasis on productivity and personal responsibility contained within state benefit schemes is thus being extended to younger older people as thresholds for expected 'retirement' from the workplace are raised.

Disability Living Allowance and Attendance Allowance

Disability Living Allowance and Attendance Allowance are both non-means-tested benefits designed to compensate for additional costs incurred through disability. Disability Living Allowance is payable to claimants under 65, and Attendance Allowance applies to claimants aged 65 and over. Both benefits can be awarded indefinitely or for a fixed period. There is an element of age discrimination here as Disability Living Allowance is a more generous allowance for a number of reasons:

- It is paid at three rather than two different rates. It includes a lower level benefit for people aged 16-65 who need help from another person for a significant portion of the day, but not frequent attention throughout the day, which is the Attendance Allowance test. There is also within the lower level of benefit an opportunity of claiming if the so-called 'cooking test' is satisfied: that the person could not cook a main meal for themselves even if they had the ingredients. So, older people are ineligible because of their age, whereas younger people would qualify.
- There is a mobility as well as a care component within Disability Living Allowance but not Attendance Allowance, which applies to those unable or virtually unable to walk. This component is not taken into account when charges for community care services are assessed, or for the assessment of care home fees contributions. However, once awarded, the mobility component continues beyond 65, with no upper age limit provided the conditions for its award continue to be met. People who receive the higher rate of Disability

Living Allowance mobility component do not have to pay road tax. Blue Badges (issued by the local authority) allow parking in restricted areas for people who are disabled.

- There is a three-month qualifying period for Disability Living Allowance, but a six-month qualifying period for Attendance Allowance. However, people who are terminally ill may apply for either benefit under the 'special rules' if they have six months or less to live.

The eligibility rules for the middle or higher rates for the care component of Disability Living Allowance are the same as those for the lower or higher rate of Attendance Allowance. The lower rate of Attendance Allowance is payable to a person who satisfies *either* the day or night conditions; the higher rate is payable to people who satisfy *both* the day and night conditions. A person will satisfy the day conditions if they are so disabled physically or mentally that, by day, they require from another person either frequent attention during the day in connection with bodily functions, or continual supervision throughout the day in order to avoid substantial danger to themselves or others. A person will satisfy the night conditions if they are so disabled physically or mentally that at night they require from another person prolonged or repeated attention in connection with bodily functions; or in order to avoid substantial danger to themselves or others, they require another person to be awake for a prolonged period or at frequent intervals for the purpose of watching over them. These definitions therefore cover both physical and mental conditions, and the need for active care as well as passive supervision. There is no requirement that there is an actual carer available to carry out these tasks and there is no requirement to account for the way in which Disability Living Allowance or Attendance Allowance is spent. Bodily functions clearly include washing, dressing and toileting, but may also include taking medication or guidance linked to sensory impairment. 'Prolonged or repeated' attention at night has been interpreted to mean attention for at least 20 minutes for at least twice a night. 'Night' is the period when the household has settled down to sleep; preparing for bed is a day-time activity.

Encouraging people to apply for Attendance Allowance and to describe the breadth of their needs is critical. Mitchell (2005) refers to a recent decision of the tribunal of social security commissioners (Case COLA 1721/2004), which answers the difficult question of whether the use of the term 'disabled' for Disability Living Allowance purposes is restricted to people with a defined medical condition, or whether it refers more generally to physical or mental impairment. The tribunal decided that the latter meaning was the correct one, in the sense of "an inability, total or partial, to perform a normal bodily or mental process"; in this case it meant that a person with learning difficulties would qualify, but in the case of older people, such a definition would be relevant to those whose functional abilities were impaired but who did not yet have a diagnosis of a specific disorder.

There is an important role for the social worker in enabling people to assess honestly the extent of their disability, and to fit it within the benefits criteria described (McDonald, 2006). People over 60 who receive Attendance Allowance or the middle or higher rate of Disability Living Allowance can use it as a 'passport' to the severe disability element of Pension Credit. It may also mean that they now qualify for disability premiums within Housing Benefit or Council Tax Benefit.

Although Attendance Allowance or Disability Living Allowance will stop entirely after 28 days in hospital or other NHS fully funded care, people who are self-funding in a care home can continue to receive Disability Living Allowance or Attendance Allowance without limit of time. Those who are supported by a local authority lose the care element (but not the mobility component) of Disability Living Allowance, or Attendance Allowance after 28 days, unless they enter into a deferred payment agreement which enables them to be treated as self-funders.

Carers Allowance

This allowance is paid to the carer, not to the person who is cared for. There is no longer an upper age limit for claiming Carers Allowance. The carer must be providing 'regular and substantial care' to one individual for at least 35 hours a week and must not earn more than £84 a week currently, from paid work. National insurance contributions will also be credited automatically towards a future state pension for the carer. The carer may themselves be in receipt of disability benefits and still qualify. However, there are some difficulties associated with the benefit:

• Under the 'overlapping benefit rules' a person may not claim Carers Allowance at the same time as some other benefits, including retirement pension. However, it may still be beneficial to make an application for Carers Allowance to establish an 'underlying entitlement' which then makes them eligible for the carers' premium within Income Support, Housing Benefit and Council Tax Benefit.

Carers Allowance will also continue for eight weeks after the death of the person being cared for.
* A major disadvantage to claiming Carers Allowance is that the person being cared for thereby loses their entitlement to the severe disability premium within Income Support or Pension Credit (which is paid at the same level).

Housing Benefit and Council Tax Benefit

Housing Benefit may be available to people on low income who have capital of less than £16,000 to cover the payment of rent, including board and lodging and hostel payments. Housing Benefit and Council Tax Benefit claimants must be 'habitually resident' in the UK and not excluded because of their immigration status. Any claim can be backdated for 12 months from the date of claim if eligibility is proved. Home owners cannot receive Housing Benefit, and will need to claim housing costs through Pension Credit. Housing Benefit will not, however, be paid on rents deemed to be 'unreasonably high' (as determined by the valuation officer) and will only be paid on the 'eligible rent', which will exclude payments for such things as heating and laundry costs and the provision of support services funded through the Supporting People programme (see page 94). Housing Benefit is not payable for those living with close relatives unless payment is on a strictly commercial basis, or the accommodation is self-contained (such as a granny flat). Council Tax Benefit is payable to the person in the household who is responsible for paying the council tax on the property. Normally non-dependant deductions are made if there is another adult living in the property because it is assumed that they contribute to the rent or council tax payment. However, if the claimant or their partner is 65 or over, the non-dependant deduction will not be applied for a period of 26 weeks. Deductions will not be made if claimants are in receipt of Attendance Allowance or the care component of Disability Living Allowance, so as not to discourage carers moving into the household. Similarly, a person who is severely mentally impaired (for example, a person with a learning difficulty or dementia) is not classed as a dependant and it will be possible to claim a deduction in council tax because of their disability. A person who lives alone is automatically entitled to a 25% deduction on Council Tax Benefit. The assessment of Housing Benefit or Council Tax Benefit takes into account both income and capital, and people over 65 have higher applicable amounts; disability premiums and carers premiums also apply. However, it is possible for a high earner with capital who is paying council tax to claim what is known as a 'second adult rebate' if a person with a low income, such as a parent who is a pensioner, lives in their household. If a person is in hospital, or moves temporarily into residential care, Housing Benefit but not Council Tax Benefit may be payable on a second home for a four-week transition period when someone is waiting to move into more suitable housing. If a person moves permanently into hospital or residential care, their unoccupied home will be totally exempt from council tax.

Charging for non-residential services

Local authorities have a power to make 'reasonable' charges for non-residential community care services under s 17 of the Health and Social Services and Social Security Adjudications Act 1983. However, if a person satisfies the authority that their means are insufficient for it to be reasonably practicable for them to pay for the service, the authority cannot require them to pay more than it is reasonably practicable for them to pay.

Although the imposition of charges for non-residential services is a power not a duty, central government funding is based on the assumption that these charges will be levied. However, s 17 does not authorise charging for services for aftercare under s 117 of the Mental Health Act 1983 (see page 84); the legal basis on which the services are provided should therefore be clarified before charges are assessed. There have historically been wide differences in policy and practice between different authorities (Baldwin and Lunt, 1996). Guidance now sets out for the first time a national framework to ensure that charging policies are fair and operate consistently. LAC (2001)32 (DH, 2001b) does not require councils to modify policies that are less favourable to users, but does require adherence to minimum standards from April 2003. These are:

* users receiving Income Support (now including Pension Credit), with a 25% 'buffer' will not be charged for services;
* users in receipt of Disability Living Allowance, Attendance Allowance or the Severe Disability Premium in Income Support should have an individual assessment of their disability-related expenditure, such as laundry, domestic help and personal assistance costs. (The mobility component of Disability Living Allowance is excluded from the assessment by the operation of s 73 of the Social Security Contributions and Benefits Act 1992);

- earnings should be disregarded as part of income;
- local authorities should provide benefits advice to enable individuals to maximise their income;
- at a minimum, the same savings limits as for residential care charges are to be applied.

The assessed charge may be challenged through the local authority's complaints procedure, or an appeal panel set up for this purpose (Clements, 2004). Arrears of charges are recoverable as a civil debt and should not involve suspension of essential services that the local authority is under a duty to provide.

User-controlled trusts

Direct payments enable money to be paid directly to the service user to pay for care (see page 30). What if the individual lacks capacity, however, and cannot control the funding themselves? In *R (A & B) v East Sussex County Council and another (no 1)* [2003] EWHC 167 (Admin), Munby J approved in principle the idea of a user independent trust to enable the family of two profoundly disabled sisters to set up a trust fund to receive and use funding for the provision of care at home. The characteristics of a legally acceptable trust in these circumstances were said to be:

- that it is a legal entity distinct from those who are to be cared for and their carers;
- that the carers do not control the company, and since they are in a minority on the board, they cannot exercise a veto;
- that the company is non-profit making and any surplus on winding up must be repaid to the council.

One further advantage of creating a user-controlled trust was highlighted in *R (on the application of Gunter) v South Western Staffordshire PCT* [2005] EWHC 1894 – that the profit margin that an independent agency would calculate on its charge for care is thereby avoided, so the end user takes the entire benefit of the funding available. Also in that case, Collins J accepted that a health care body (in this case the PCT) could also contract with a user-controlled trust to provide health care services using its powers under Schedule 5A of the NHS Act 1977.

Paying for residential care

The following general principles apply to the assessment of charges for residential accommodation that local authorities have a duty to levy under s 22 of the National Assistance Act 1948. Department of Health Guidance is amended on a yearly basis by the Charging for Residential Accommodation Guide (CRAG) to which reference should be made for the most recent updates. Current guidance is contained in LAC (2006)12, CRAG amendment No 25 (DH, 2006d).

Fees are charged at the 'standard rate', or full cost to the local authority, unless after means-testing a lower contribution is levied, leaving aside a Personal Expenses Allowance for the resident. Local authorities, however, have a discretion to charge less than the standard rate for short-term care of up to 8 weeks.

- Residents are to be assessed on their own income and capital. There is no legal requirement for a spouse to disclose their income or assets. If the local authority wishes to enforce a contribution from a 'liable relative', a power likely to be removed by statute in the near future, they can take proceedings in the magistrates' court if no voluntary arrangement can be made.
- The value of an unsold property is not taken into account for the first three months, and for permanent residents is not counted at all when a spouse or partner, or a relative over the age of 60 or a child under 16, or someone who is disabled remains living there. There is discretion in other cases. Where property is jointly owned, it is the market value of the resident's share that is taken into account; where no separation of the property is possible, this will be minimal.
- Self-funding residents are entitled to claim Attendance Allowance or Disability Living Allowance (see page 127) to help meet care costs. This also applies to the period before a property is sold when the resident might be receiving interim public funding.
- Local authorities may enter into deferred payment agreements whereby a property is sold only on the resident's death and no earlier interest accrues. Where such an agreement is entered into, residents may top up fees from their own capital (ss 53-55 of the Health and Social Care Act 2001). The local authority can also, without consent, impose a legal charge on property to recoup a debt.
- Third party contributions may be available to enable residents to choose a place in a home that is more expensive than the local authority's usual maximum cost.

- Local authorities cannot be charged for the nursing care element of care homes with nursing and nor can residents, but residents who pay their own fees can choose to refuse NHS funding (Easterbrook, 2005).
- People who receive accommodation under s 117 of the Mental Health Act 1983 cannot be charged for any element of that accommodation.
- People who had 'preserved rights' before 31 March 1993, when social security funding was transferred to local authorities, are now the responsibility of the local authority in which they are ordinarily resident.
- If it is shown that a resident has deliberately deprived themselves of capital to reduce a charge for accommodation, the local authority can seek reimbursement of 'notional capital' under the provisions of s 22 of the Health and Social Services and Social Security Adjudications Act 1983, but only if intent can be proved. In *R (Beeson) v Dorset County Council* [2002] EWCA Civ 1812 a high evidential threshold was set for showing that the resident's transfer of property to his son was done with the intention of avoiding care home fees. Bankruptcy proceedings can also be instigated. For a transfer within six months of entering residential care, assets can be traced into the hands of recipients under s 21 of the above Act.

For independent sector homes, the contract to pay for care is between the local authority and the home owner; this remains the case even when the resident pays their proportion of the fees directly to the proprietor. Residents should be given a written explanation of how their charges are worked out and should be monitored by the local authority for financial support when they approach the capital limit (currently £21,500) below which the local authority will contribute to charges on a sliding scale. (DH, 1996). People who receive a savings credit under the Pension Credit rules receive a small weekly disregard to protect former savings. Where a spouse remains at home, an occupational or private pension can be divided on a 50/50 basis for the benefit of both.

Case study 4: Finance

Harold Beddowes is 73 years old and lives alone in a bungalow that he owns. Harold receives basic state pension and an occupational pension of £20 per week. Harold has no close relatives except for a niece, Thelma, aged 55, who visits him every other day. Thelma also works part time in a local pub. Harold has recently been diagnosed with Alzheimer's Disease, and is reliant on Thelma to do his shopping and cleaning. Thelma also takes his laundry and prepares meals for the freezer for the days when she is not able to visit. Money is very tight, and although Thelma would like to continue to visit Harold as often as she does, she has now been offered longer hours at the pub. Harold would like to be able to pay Thelma for doing daily tasks for him, but at present is not able to do so.

What advice can you give to both Harold and Thelma to help them to decide whether the income that each has can be increased by claiming more benefits?

Thelma also collects Harold's pension each week and helps him to deal with all his financial affairs. Harold is becoming less able to keep track of the bills that need to be paid and of the money in his bank account. Ideally, Thelma would like to deal with everything herself, as she finds that dealing with financial matters makes Harold very anxious. Harold's condition appears to be deteriorating and he is beginning to talk to Thelma about planning for a move into permanent residential care.

Consider the various legal devices that exist for dealing with someone else's financial affairs and discuss their appropriateness in this case.

Further reading

Letts, P. (1998) *Managing other people's money*, London: Age Concern. This is a practical and useful book which describes the working of powers of attorney and of the Court of Protection specifically in respect of older people.

Lush, D. and Cretney, S. (2001) *Cretney and Lush on enduring powers of attorney* (5th edn), Bristol: Jordans.
The leading legal textbook on enduring powers of attorney, describing the law in England and Wales.

Heywood, N., Lush, D. and Massey, A. (2001) *Heywood and Massey: Court of Protection practice* (13th edn), London: Sweet and Maxwell.
The latest edition of the classic work on the Court of Protection for reference.

Greaves, I. (published annually) *Disability rights handbook*, London: Disability Alliance.
A guide to benefits and services for disabled people, their families and carers.

FIVE

Death and family provision

Having organised one's business affairs through life, it is equally important to ensure that clear arrangements are made to deal with such matters on death. There are many popular misconceptions about who gets what and how the system works.

Whatever the position in life, all management arrangements cease on death. An attorney's authority automatically ends, a Court of Protection receivership ceases (save for the formal winding-up of the court proceedings) and assets and liabilities become the responsibility of the duly constituted personal representatives. Arguments that "I am the next-of-kin" are irrelevant.

Funeral arrangements

Disposal of the body is the immediate problem. If the coroner is involved, as they will be in sudden or unexpected deaths, then the body is subject to their jurisdiction and no funeral can be held until they agree to release it, having been satisfied that it is not needed for further tests. Every NHS hospital should have a procedure for dealing with the death of patients, respecting their cultural and religious beliefs (Easterbrook, 2005). The NHS will arrange a funeral for a person who dies in hospital who has no family to do so; otherwise the local authority has power to do so under the Public Health (Control of Disease) Act 1984 (Easterbrook, 2005).

Strictly, the funeral arrangements should be the responsibility of the executors if there is a will. Often, family or friends make the arrangements and then tell the executors; however, they should not be surprised if some professional executors object to arrangements to which they have not been a party. As a matter of contract law, the person who makes the arrangements with the funeral director is the one who is responsible for payment of the bill – the contract is between those two parties. If the estate does not pay, the funeral director will have a contractual claim against whoever made the arrangements for payment.

If there is little money, or the death is sudden or occurs in complex circumstances, a number of issues will need to be considered. In the former case, the Department for Work and Pensions may pick up the bill if the deceased had few assets but only if the person making the arrangements is on means-tested benefits (see page 124). Even so, any assets that there may be in the estate are looked to in order to repay the Department for Work and Pensions' outlay. While funeral arrangements may be mentioned in a will, they are only an expression of wishes and not legally binding on the family or executors. Practical considerations may make the wishes impossible to carry out. Nowadays increasing numbers of people take out prepaid funeral plans and it is wise to investigate their possible existence. Most plans are tied to the use of a nominated funeral director. The cost of a memorial can also be a cause of contention. Again the contract is between the person who places the order and the monumental mason. Unless express provision is made for meeting the cost from the estate it is not a debt that has to be paid from the estate, ahead of the beneficiaries. Limitations may be placed on what the memorial can consist of depending on local authority or church regulations for particular graveyards.

The death has to be registered before the funeral can take place. If the coroner is involved, it can be registered afterwards if the coroner has authorised the funeral and there is no inquest, or it is done automatically after any inquest verdict. The closest available kin must perform the registration; if there is no kin, whoever is arranging the funeral or the householder of the premises where the death took place may find themselves involved.

Coroners

There are currently over 500,000 deaths in England and Wales per year and two fifths of these are formally reported to the coroner before authority is given to release the body. Overall responsibility for coroners' enquiries and inquests lies with the Department for Constitutional Affairs in accordance with the Coroners Act 1988 and the Coroners Rules 1984. The statistics indicate a high workload and complex issues; in 2004 (DCA, 2006) 28,300 inquests took place, of which 570 were with a jury. A death must be reported to the coroner where the cause or circumstances of the death are unknown, or if the death happened during the course of an operation, or the patient had not been seen by the certifying doctor within the 14 days preceding death. The coroner will then decide whether a post-mortem is needed. The coroner's office will need to know if this process should be expedited, perhaps for religious reasons (Easterbrook, 2005). The Human Tissues Act 2004 governs the use of human tissues and organs following a post-mortem, but the basic rule is that organs and tissue removed should be returned to the body unless permission has been given for transplants.

An inquest is held where there is reasonable cause to suspect that there has been a violent or unnatural death, or the deceased has died in public custody or from certain notifiable diseases. When the death has occurred in prison or police custody or "in circumstances the continuance or possible recurrence of which is prejudicial to the health or safety of the public or any section of the public" (s 8(3)(d) of the Coroners Act 1988), a jury is required. The inquest is a public court proceeding but is inquisitorial rather than adversarial; its primary purpose is to find facts rather than to attribute blame or liability. A review of the system of death certification and investigation (Luce, 2003) recommended that professional health care staff, members of the care inspectorate, funeral directors and family members should be able to refer cases to the coroner. This was in part a response to the Harold Shipman Inquiry with which it was contemporaneous. Family members, it was recommended, should be more involved in the process and supported through it, by legal representation if necessary. Legislation is anticipated to introduce national standards and further training for coroners (DCA, 2006).

In *McCann v UK* (1998) 28 EHRR 245, the 'Death on the Rock' case in which British security forces were involved, the European Court of Human Rights interpreted the state's obligations under Article 2 of the Convention as requiring an effective public investigation by an independent official body whenever 'agents of the State' were implicated in a death. The House of Lords has interpreted the obligation to investigate as applying not only to individual fault (as in *McCann*), but to what is described as 'systemic neglect' (*R v HM Coroner for the County of West Yorkshire ex parte Sacker and R v HM Coroner for the Western District of Somerset, ex parte Middleton* [2004] All ER (D) 268). Where an inquest is held, the decision of the jury in s 11(5)(b) of the Coroners Act 1988 as to 'how' the deceased died is thus not simply to be interpreted as 'by what means', but 'in what circumstances', allowing "a judgemental conclusion of a factual nature" (para 37) that meets the expectations of the next of kin. The decision in *Middleton* means that, even without reform of the Coroners Act itself, inquests may now be required to include a detailed and critical examination of the events leading up to a death that occurs in circumstances giving cause for concern. Although the inquest does not, as such, attribute blame for the purpose of further legal actions, it has enabled a 'narrative verdict' to be delivered that more fully explains the circumstances and antecedents of the death than 'closed' verdicts, which focus on categorisation rather than causation.

Some of the recent cases have explored the scope of the coroner's inquest in relation to the death of people receiving care in hospital, and a more conservative approach to Article 2 has been shown. In *R (on the application of Takoushis) v Inner London North Coroner and another* [2005] EWCA Civ 1440, a voluntary psychiatric patient given leave to visit the day hospital disappeared and was found preparing to jump off Tower Bridge. He was taken to a hospital Accident and Emergency department but absconded and was later seen to jump into the River Thames. It was held that the holding of an inquest together with the possibility of civil and criminal proceedings was sufficient in a case where medical negligence was alleged to satisfy the requirements of Article 2 of the European Convention. Unlike the cases of death in police custody, the system did not have to provide for an investigation by the state, although the widow was seeking an inquiry into the death. In the case of *R (on the application of Goodson) v Bedfordshire and Luton Coroner* [2004] EWHC 2931, the claimant's father had died unexpectedly in an NHS hospital following elective surgery. The claimant asked that the inquest should be conducted as an 'inquiry' for the purposes of Article 2 and that an independent medical witness should be instructed for that purpose. Both applications were refused and a simple verdict of death by misadventure returned. A distinction was drawn between the effectiveness overall of the state's establishment of a framework for legal protection (as here), and the exceptional cases where there was a possible breach of the state's own positive obligation to protect life and where a separate procedural obligation under Article 2 would arise. It seems therefore that the ordinary legal system is seen as sufficient compliance with Article 2 in most cases of medical negligence, although there is arguably potential for development of the procedural obligation where the patient is detained, for example, under the Mental Health Act 1983 or other compulsory intervention.

Distribution of estate

Most joint assets can be transferred fairly easily to the surviving co-owner or owners simply on production of a death certificate. That is because the property is held on what is known as a 'joint tenancy', whereby the property passes automatically to the surviving co-owner or owners. Assets held this way cannot be controlled by a will as, by operation of law, the document controlling the joint ownership is the conveyance on house purchase, or application form to open an account, and it takes precedence over the dispositions in a will.

One exception to this is where land is owned by co-owners on a 'tenancy in common' basis. In that instance, the surviving co-owners have the title in their names and can dispose of it (although one surviving co-owner will have to appoint a second person as trustee before a purchaser will pay over the purchase price). In this case the land is held for the estate of the deceased co-owner and the survivors in the relevant proportions on which it was originally held. A 'tenancy in common' can be applied to other assets but banks and building societies have difficulty recognising the concept in practice.

Assets in the sole name of the deceased become temporarily frozen once the death certificate is produced. It is for the personal representatives to deal with these assets once they can establish their right so to do. The broad guideline is that if the total estate is worth over £15,000 then either probate or letters of administration (a grant of representation) is needed: if the estate value is less than £15,000 then neither is necessary. Even so, it can sometimes work out simpler, and marginally cheaper in practice, to obtain probate or letters of administration for a small estate if there are several tiny assets in different places; the grant of representation is universally acceptable, whereas each bank, building society or insurance company has its own slightly different procedure when no grant is available.

A will should ensure that the deceased's wishes are carried out and those whom the deceased wished to benefit receive their due. The will must conform with the formalities of the Wills Act 1837 (as amended), for example that it is in writing, signed and witnessed by two independent witnesses and that all three signatures take place together and in the right order.

Although it is tempting to try writing out one's will oneself, or to buy a will form from a stationer, some of the formalities are often missed out, and the 'will' fails and so has no legal effect. This is often not discovered until after the person has died, by which time it is too late to rectify the mistakes unless everyone involved is prepared to agree and has legal capacity.

Most wills, if professionally drawn, are certainly not expensive relative to the overall value of the estate and the importance of directing the inheritance to the right place. For some small estates it may be possible for people over the age of 70 or with a terminal condition to make wills by way of Public Funding (Legal Aid) if they can come within the means-tested limits. Ownership of one's home is ignored.

If there is no will, the estate is distributed according to set rules laid down by the Administration of Estates Act 1925 and subsequent statutory instruments. Everything does not automatically pass to a surviving spouse or civil partner, or to the eldest son on the death of both or the second parent. In each case, both the size of the deceased's estate and the classes of relatives they have left are considered. A civil partner now has the same inheritance rights as a spouse.

If there is a spouse/civil partner and no children, the spouse/civil partner inherits personal chattels, the first £200,000 and half the rest of the estate over £200,000 provided they survive the deceased by 28 days. The other half passes to the deceased's other relatives, for example parents or brothers and sisters.

If there is a spouse/civil partner and children of the deceased, then the surviving spouse/civil partner receives personal chattels, the; first £125,000 and the income only from half the estate over £125,000 provided they survive the deceased by 28 days. The other half passes immediately to the deceased's children at age 18, as does the first half on the death of the surviving spouse/civil partner.

If there is no spouse or civil partner, the whole estate is distributed among all members of the nearest class of relatives to the deceased, beginning with children or other issue; if there are no children then it falls to parents, then brothers and sisters and so on. If having looked as far as cousins, there are no relatives, the entire estate can end up going to the state (that is, going into government coffers).

Family provision

It is always open to people who feel that the deceased has not provided for them adequately to contest the will or operation of the intestacy rules by suing the estate under the Inheritance (Provision for Family and Dependants) Act 1975. To bring a successful action, the claimant must come within one of five classes of people able to sue: spouses, ex-spouses, children, children of a marriage (basically step-children) and any other person. This last class is most commonly used by surviving partners of a non-marital or same-sex but not a civil partnership relationship where, if they can show they have been living together for at least two years, then a successful claim is no longer as difficult to bring as it used to be. Otherwise, the claimant must show some form of dependency: for example, if an adult child, making their own way in the world, challenges a parent's will that leaves everything to charity, they will most certainly not succeed.

Often one spouse/civil partner will make a will cutting out or restricting the inheritance of their partner who is in care, in the belief that the state system will fund them. There is a suggestion that local authorities and the Department for Work and Pensions will encourage such surviving spouses to bring actions under this Act on the basis that they have not been provided for adequately. Only time will tell how much this provision will be used, but families should be aware of the potential difficulties if one spouse makes a will totally cutting out their partner on that partner's admission into permanent residential care which is heavily subsidised by the state. The counter argument is that a surviving spouse, particularly if female, is in receipt of increased pensions as a result of the death and so provision has been made in that way. The question then becomes, is it adequate?

In *Cunliffe v Fielden and another* [2006] 2 All ER 115, the wife of the deceased challenged an order for the payment of a lump sum of £800,000 out of his estate of £1.4 million under s 3(2) of the 1975 Act. The court was required to have regard to the provision that the applicant might reasonably have expected to receive if the marriage had been terminated by divorce and not death. However, it was held that, considering the brevity of the marriage and the limited nature of the widow's contribution, the provision should not be of a level or of a nature to enable her to remain for the rest of her life in the former matrimonial home or at the standard of living which she had enjoyed during the marriage. It could also take into account the capital she had received by way of survivorship as well as income from employment. This was less than she had been left in the will and less than she would have received according to the principle of equality after divorce, as the deceased spouse was required only to make 'reasonable provision'; he could dispose of his estate as he wished otherwise.

Taxation

No Capital Gains Tax is payable on death. The death duty tax is Inheritance Tax. Gifts between husband and wife and civil partners (but not cohabitees, although this is likely to change) are exempt from tax, unless the receiving spouse or civil partner is non-UK domiciled, so that any amount can pass from one to the other, tax-free. Gifts to charities are also exempt.

Subject to reliefs for business or agricultural property, tax is paid after the first £285,000 (from April 2006) at a flat rate of 40%. This figure is due to rise to £300,000 in 2007. The size of the estate is calculated by looking at the assets left on death, those given away in the last seven years immediately preceding death and any trust funds in which the deceased had a right to income. Also taken into account is the value of the deceased's share of assets that have passed by survivorship on a joint tenancy basis to someone else. Debts, funeral bills and so on are deducted, and the resultant net figure is the taxable estate.

It is possible to save tax by husband and wife equalising their estates – seeing that they each have assets of roughly equivalent value – and then making gifts down to the next generation on the first death or creating a discretionary trust of the tax-free band on the first death, rather than leaving it all to the survivor. It is worth taking professional advice to ensure the correct steps are taken.

After death, deeds of variation can be entered into, altering the dispositions of a will or the operation of the intestacy rules. These are often done for tax-saving purposes and, as long as everyone agrees, the document is written and entered into within two years of death, it should be acceptable to the Inland Revenue. However, it is better to have planned beforehand than to rely on a post-death variation to save the day.

Case study 5: Inheritance

Jacob Jenkins, a retired solicitor, has lived alone for many years. Two years ago he employed a housekeeper, Ruth Evans. In addition to paying her a salary, Jacob has bought Ruth an expensive car and has given her power of attorney over all his financial affairs. Jacob has made a will leaving a small bequest to charity and the residue of his estate to Ruth. Jacob's two nephews (his only living relatives) are concerned about this. They see their uncle twice a year, on his birthday and at Christmas, but are shocked at the extent to which he appears to have deteriorated both physically and mentally since their last visit six months ago. They say that their uncle has spoken to them about wanting to sell the house to go into residential care, but he has also said that Ruth won't allow him to do this. They feel that Ruth is exploiting their uncle and are concerned to know what the legal issues are in this situation.

Further reading

'What to do after a death', DSS leaflet D49

'What to do when someone dies', Consumers Association

Ashton, G. and Edis, A. (2004) *Elderly client handbook* (3rd edn), London: Law Society.
Published in association with Solicitors for the Elderly, this guide to practice with elderly clients is an administrative technical handbook for solicitors.

Battison, T. (2000) *The understanding bereavement training pack*, London: Age Concern.
A guide for carers working with older people covering good practice when dealing with death, mourning, rituals, customs, support of relatives, colleagues and friends.

Conclusion

The previous chapters of this book have looked at the needs of older people in the community, in residential care and in hospital settings, and have considered both personal and financial issues. The position of carers and other family members has also been recognised, and guidance has been given on dealing with the formalities of death and administering an estate. The intention has been to show the relevance of legal knowledge at each stage in this process. The importance of assessing needs holistically has also been emphasised in a way that aims to facilitate both inter-agency and inter-professional working. So, too, this book can give a broadly based account of legal issues, helping other professionals to see situations in legal terms. More specialist legal advice will, however, often be needed to take forward these issues, and a list of organisations relevant to older people is contained in the Appendix.

Some solicitors will also specialise in giving advice to older clients (look for members of Solicitors for the Elderly) or will be members of the Law Society's probate section or mental health panel. Communication is made easier if other professionals are able to pick out key themes or words, such as 'incapacity' or 'consent' that have a meaning for lawyers in order to structure inter-professional dialogues. It is hoped that that this book has given social workers in particular the vocabulary with which to conceptualise in legal terms some of the issues with which their clients are faced.

There is as yet unrealised potential for using rights-based arguments to challenge the social exclusion of older people (Thompson, 1995). This means that older people should be seen not as passive recipients of services, but as directly involved in service planning and design and with a constructive role to play in challenging service standards and delivery. The Human Rights Act 1998 is likely to be important in ensuring the protection of dignity and choice, in the absence of any direct national legislation outside the employment field that outlaws discrimination against older people. Again, seeing issues such as the rationing of health and social care in legal terms will enable challenges to be made which look not only at procedural propriety (important though this is), but also at the quantification of basic levels of service. One of the most important changes that still needs to take place is the development of positive duties to support rights, particularly for people who are vulnerable through mental disorder or incapacity. Advocacy from others is important in ensuring that their voices are heard, and lawyers and social workers working in partnership can do much to achieve this.

List of organisations

Action on Elder Abuse
    Astral House
    1268 London Road
    Norbury
    London
    SW16 4ER
    Tel: 020 8765 7000
    www.elderabuse.org.uk

Age Concern Cymru
    Units 13 and 14
    Neptune Court
    Vanguard Way
    Cardiff
    CF24 SPJ
    Tel: 029 2043 1555
    www.accymru.org.uk

Age Concern England
    1268 London Road
    London
    SW16 4ER
    Tel: 020 8765 7200
    www.ageconcern.org.uk

Alzheimer's Society
    Gordon House
    10 Greencoat Place
    London
    SW1P 1PH
    Tel: 0845 300 0336
    www.alzheimers.org.uk

British Association of Social Workers
  16 Kent Street
  Birmingham
  B5 6RD
  Tel: 0121 622 3911
  www.basw.co.uk

British Medical Association
  BMA House
  Tavistock Square
  London
  WC1H 9JH
  Tel: 020 7387 4499
  www.bma.org.uk

British Association/College of Occupational Therapists
  106-114 Borough High Street
  London
  SE1 1LB
  Tel: 020 7357 7480
  www.cot.co.uk

Carers UK
  Ruth Pitter House
  20-25 Glasshouse Yard
  London
  EC1A 4JT
  Tel: 020 7490 8824
  www.carersonline.org.uk

Child Poverty Action Group
  94 White Lion Street
  London
  N1 9FP
  Tel: 020 7837 7979
  www.cpag.org.uk

Citizens Advice
  115-123 Pentonville Road
  London
  N1 9LZ
  Tel: 020 7833 2181
  www.citizensadvice.org.uk

Commission for Patient and Public Involvement in Health
  7th Floor
  120 Edmund Street
  Birmingham
  B3 2ES
  Tel: 0845 120 7111
  www.cppih.org

Commission for Social Care Inspection
  33 Greycoat Street
  London
  SW1P 2QF
  Tel: 0845 015 0120
  www.csci.org.uk

Counsel and Care
  Twyman House
  16 Bonny Street
  London
  NW1 9PG
  Tel: 020 7241 8555
  www.counselandcare.org.uk

Disability Alliance
  Universal House
  88-94 Wentworth Street
  London
  E1 75A
  Tel: 020 7247 8776
  www.disabilityalliance.org

General Medical Council
  178 Great Portland Street
  London
  W1W 5JE
  Tel: 020 7915 3603
  www.gmc-uk.org

General Social Care Council
  Goldings House
  2 Hays Lane
  London
  SE1 2HB
  Tel: 020 7397
  www.gscc.org.uk

Healthcare Commission
  FREEPOST NAT 18958
  Complaints Investigation Team
  Manchester
  M1 9XZ
  Tel: 0845 601 3012
  www.healthcarecommission.org.uk

Health Professions Council
  Park House
  184 Kennington Park Road
  London
  SE11 4BU
  Tel: 020 7582 0866
  www.hpc-uk.org

Health Service Ombudsman
  Millbank Tower
  Millbank
  London
  SW1P 4QP
  Tel: 0845 015 4033
  www.ombudsman.org.uk

Help the Aged
  207–221 Pentonville Road
  London
  N1 9VZ
  Tel: 0808 800 6565
  www.helptheaged.org.uk

King's Fund
  11–13 Cavendish Square
  London
  W1G 0AN
  Tel: 020 7307 2400
  www.kingsfund.org.uk

Law Society
  113 Chancery Lane
  London
  WC2A 1PL
  Tel: 020 7242 1222
  www.lawsociety.org.uk

Local Government Association
  Local Government House
  Smith Square
  London
  SW1P 3HZ
  Tel: 020 7664 3131
  www.lga.gov.uk

Mind
  15–19 Broadway
  London
  E15 4BQ
  Tel: 020 8519 2122
  www.mind.org.uk

National Association of Widows
  48 Queens Road
  Coventry
  CV1 3EH
  Tel: 024 7663 4646
  www.nawidows.org.uk

National Patient Safety Agency
  4–8 Maple Street
  London
  W1T 5HD
  Tel: 020 7927 9500
  www.npsa.nhs.uk

RADAR: The disability network
  12 City Forum
  250 City Road
  London
  EC1V 8AF
  Tel: 020 7250 3222
  www.radar.org.uk

Royal National Institute for Deaf People
  19–23 Featherstone Street
  London
  EC1Y 8SL
  Tel: 0808 808 9000
  www.rnid.org.uk

Royal National Institute for the Blind
  105 Judd Street
  London
  WC1H 9NE
  Tel: 0845 766 9999
  www.rnib.org.uk

Shelter
  88 Old Street
  London
  EC1V 9HV
  Tel: 020 7505 2169
  www.shelternet.org.uk

Social Care Institute for Excellence
  1st Floor
  Goldings House
  2 Hays Lane
  London
  SE1 2HB
  Tel: 020 7089 6840
  www.scie.org.uk

Solicitors for the Elderly Ltd
  PO Box 257
  Broxbourne
  Hertfordshire
  EN10 7YY
  Tel: 01992 471568
  www.solicitorsfortheelderly.com

The Relatives & Residents Association
  24 The Ivories
  6–18 Northampton Street
  London
  NI1 2HY
  Tel: 020 7359 8148
  www.relres.org.uk

United Kingdom Home Care Association
  42b Banstead Road
  Carshalton Beeches
  Surrey
  SM5 3NW
  Tel: 020 8288 1551
  www.ukhca.co.uk

Womens Royal Voluntary Service
  Garden House
  Milton Hall
  Steventon
  Abingdon
  Oxfordshire
  OX13 6AD
  Tel: 01235 442900
  www.wrvs.org.uk

References

ADSS (Association of Directors of Social Services) (2003) *Inverting the triangle of care*, London: ADSS.

ADSS (2005) *Safeguarding Adults: A National Framework of Standards for good practice and outcomes in adult protection work*, London: ADSS.

Age Concern (2004) *Some basic facts*, London: Age Concern.

Age Concern (2006a) 'Advance statements, advance directives and living wills', Information Sheet 5, London: Age Concern.

Age Concern (2006b) 'Fact sheet no 19 on state pensions', London: Age Concern.

Age Concern/University of Kent (2005) *How ageist is Britain?*, London: Age Concern.

Aldridge, J. and Becker, S. (1993) *Children who care: Inside the world of young carers*, Loughborough: Department of Social Sciences, Loughborough University.

Arden, A. and Hunter, C. (2003) *Manual of housing law* (7th edn), London: Thompson, Sweet and Maxwell.

Arksey, H., Hepworth, D. and Quereshi, H. (2000) *Carer's needs and the Carers Act*, York: Social Policy Research Unit, University of York.

Ashton, G. and Edis, A. (2004) *Elderly client handbook* (3rd edn), London: Law Society.

Audit Commission (2000a) *Fully equipped: The provision of equipment to older or disabled people by the NHS and social services in England and Wales*, London: Audit Commission.

Audit Commission (2000b) *Forget me not: Developing mental health services for older people in England*, London: Audit Commission.

Audit Commission (2002) *Forget me not 2002: Developing mental health services for older people in England*, London: Audit Commission.

Audit Commission, Health Care Commission and Commission for Social Care Inspection (2006) *Living well in later life*, London: Audit Commission.

Baldwin, S. and Lunt, N. (1996) *Charging ahead: Development of local authority charging policies for community care*, Bristol: The Policy Press.

Ball, C. and McDonald, A. (2003) *Law for social workers* (4th edn), London: Ashgate.

Bamford, T. (2001) *Commissioning and purchasing*, London: Routledge/Community Care.

Bartlett, P. and Sandland, R. (2003) *Mental health law: Policy and practice* (2nd edn), Oxford: Oxford University Press.

Battison, T. (2000) *The understanding bereavement training pack*, London: Age Concern.

BBA (British Bankers' Association) (2005) *Banking for mentally incapacitated customers*, London: BBA.

Bielanska, C. (2004) 'Care home contracts', *New Law Journal*, vol 154, pp 1565-70.

BMA (British Medical Association) (2001) *Consent toolkit*, London: BMA.

BMA (2002) *Decisions relating to cardiopulmonary resuscitation,* London: BMA.

BMA and Law Society (2004) *Assessment of mental capacity – Guidance for doctors and lawyers* (2nd edn), London: BMA and the Law Society.

Bradley, G. and Manthorpe, J. (1995) 'The dilemmas of financial assessment, professional and ethical difficulties', *Practice*, vol 7, no 4.

Braye, S. and Preston-Shoot, M. with Cull, L.-A., Johns, R. and Roche, J. (2005) *Teaching, learning and assessment in law in social work education*, London: SCIE.

British Institute of Human Rights (2002) *Something for everyone: The impact of the Human Rights Act and the need for a Human Rights Commission*, London, BIHR.

Cafferkey, A. (2005) 'Housing law update', *New Law Journal*, vol 155, no 7201, 18 November.

Clark, H., Gough, H. and Macfarlane, A. (2004) *It pays dividends: Direct payments and older people*, Bristol/York: The Policy Press/Joseph Rowntree Foundation.

Clements, L. (2004) *Community care and the law* (3rd edn), London: Legal Action Group.

Cornes, M. and Clough, R. (2004) 'Inside multi-disciplinary practice: challenges for single assessment', *Journal of Integrated Care*, vol 12, no 2, pp 18-29.

CSCI (Commission for Social Care Inspection) (2005) *Leaving hospital – Revisited*, London: CSCI.

CSCI (2006) *Real voices, real choices: The qualities people expect from care services*, London: CSCI.

CSCI (2006a) *Adult performance indicators for 2006-07*, London: CSCI.

Dawson, C. (2000) *Independent successes: Implementing direct payments*, York: Joseph Rowntree Foundation.

Dawson, C. and McDonald, A. (2000) 'Assessing mental capacity: A checklist for social workers', *Practice* vol 12, no 2, pp 5-20.

Day, P., Klein, R. and Redmayne, S. (1996) *Why regulate? Regulating residential care for elderly people*, Bristol: The Policy Press.

DCA (Department of Constitutional Affairs) (2006) *Reform of the coroner system: Briefing note*, London: DCA.

DCLG (Department for Communities and Local Government) (2006) *Homelessness code of guidance for local authorities*, London: Homelessness and Housing Support Directorate.

DH (Department of Health) (1990) *Community care in the next decade and beyond*, London: DH.

DH (1991a) *Care management and assessment: Practitioners' guide*, London: DH.

DH (1991b) *The right to complain*, London: DH.

DH (1993a) *Approvals and directions for arrangements from 1 April 1993 made under section 8 to the NHS Act 1977 and sections 21 and 29 of the National Assistance Act 1948*, LAC (93)10, London: DH.

DH (1993b) *Ordinary residence*, LAC (93)7, London: DH.

DH (1995a) *Young carers*, CI (95)12, London: DH.

DH (1995b) *NHS responsibilities for meeting continuing health care needs*, HSG (95)8, London: DH.

DH (1996) *Charges for residential accommodation: CRAG amendment number 15*, LAC (2001)25, London: DH.

DH (1997a) *The new NHS: Modern, dependable*, London: DH.

DH (1997b) *Responsibilities of local authority social services departments implications of recent legal judgements*, LASSL (97)13, London: DH.

DH (1998a) *Modernising social services*, Cm 4169, London: DH.

DH (1998b) *Community Care (Residential Accommodation) Act 1998*, LAC (98)19, London: DH.

DH (1998c) *The transfer of frail older NHS patients to other long stay settings*, HSC 1998/048, London: DH.

DH (1999) *Review of the Mental Health Act 1983: Report of the Expert Committee*, London: DH.

DH (2000a) *Practitioners' guide to carers assessment under the Carers and Disabled Children Act 2000*, London: DH.

DH (2000b) *No secrets: Guidance on developing and implementing multi-agency policies and procedures to protect vulnerable adults*, London: DH.

DH (2000c) *Listening to people*, LASSL (2000)7, London: DH.

DH (2001a) *National service framework for older people*, London: DH.

DH (2001b) *Fair charging policies for home care and other non-residential social services*, LAC (2001)32, London: DH.

DH (2001c) *Community equipment services*, LAC (2001)13, London: DH.

DH (2001d) *Carers and Disabled Children Act 2000: Carers and people with parental responsibility for disabled children: Policy guidance*, London: DH.

DH (2001e) *Intermediate care*, LAC (2001)1, London: DH.

DH (2001f) *Continuing care: NHS and local councils' responsibilities*, LAC (2001)18, London: DH.

DH (2001g) *Guidance on free nursing care in nursing homes*, HSC (2001)17, London: DH.

DH (2002a) *Fair access to care services: Guidance on eligibility criteria for adult social care*, London: DH.

DH (2002b) *The single assessment process*, London: DH.

DH (2002c) *Developing services for carers and families of people with mental illness*, London: DH.

DH (2002d) *Care management for older people with serious mental problems*, London: DH.

DH (2003a) *Community care services for carers and children's services (direct payments) guidance England*, London: DH.

DH (2003b) *Changes to local authorities charging regime for community equipment and intermediate care services*, LAC (2003)14, London: DH.

DH (2003c) *Discharge from hospital: Pathway, process and practice*, London: DH.

DH (2003d) *The NHS end of life care programme*, London: DH.

DH (2003e) *Care homes for older people: National minimum standards and the Care Homes Regulations* (3rd edn), London: DH.

DH (2003f) *End of life care initiative*, London: DH.

DH (2004a) *Choosing health: Making healthy choices easier*, Cm 6374, Norwich: The Stationery Office

DH (2004b) *The community care assessment directions 2004*, LAC (2004)24, London: DH.

DH (2004c) *Government response to the House of Commons Health Committee report on palliative care, Fourth report of session 2003-04*, Cm 6327, London: DH.

DH (2004d) *Learning from complaints*, London: DH.

DH (2004e) *Better health in old age*, London: DH.

DH (2004f) *Guidance on National Assistance Act 1948 (Choice of Accommodation) Directions 1992 and National Assistance (Residential Accommodation) (Additional Payments and Assessment of Resources) (Amendment) (England) Regulations 2001, LAC (2004) 20*, London: DH.

DH (2005a) *Independence, well-being and choice: Our vision for the future of social care for adults in England and Wales*, Cm 6499, London: DH.

DH (2005b) *Ensuring that all recipients of high band NHS-funded nursing care have been correctly considered against eligibility criteria for fully funded NHS continuing care*, London: DH.

DH (2005c) *Bournewood Consultation: The approach to be taken in response to the judgement of the European Court of Human Rights in the 'Bournewood' case*, London: DH.

DH (2006a) *Our health, our care, our say: A new direction for community services*, London: DH.

DH (2006b) *A new ambition for old age: Next steps in implementing the national service framework for older people*, London: DH.

DH (2006c) *NHS continuing health care: Action following the Grogan Judgement*, London: DH.

DH (2006d) *Charges for residential accommodation: CRAG amendment No 25*, LAC (2006)12: London: DH.

DH (2006e) *Explanatory memorandum to the Local Authority Social Services Complaints (England) Regulations 2006, SI 2006/1681*, London: DH.

Dickens, J. (2004) 'Risks and responsibilities – the role of the local authority lawyer in child care cases', *Child and Family Law Quarterly*, vol 16, no 1, pp 1-14.

DWP (Department for Work and Pensions) (2006a) *Security in retirement: Towards a new pensions system*, London: DWP.

DWP (2006b) *A new deal for welfare: Empowering people to work*, Cm 6730, London: DWP.

Easterbrook, L. (2003) *Moving on from community care: The treatment, care and support of older people in England*, London: Age Concern.

Easterbrook, L. (2005) *Your rights to health care*, London: Age Concern.

Glasby, J. and Littlechild, P. (2004) *The health and social care divide*, Bristol: The Policy Press.

GMC (General Medical Council) (2002) *Withholding and withdrawing life-prolonging medical treatment: Good practice in decision making,* London: GMC.

Gorman, H. and Postle, K. (2003) *Transforming community care: A distorted vision?*, London: BASW.

GSCC (General Social Care Council) (2002) *Code of practice for social care workers*, London: GSCC.

Ham, C. (2004) *Health policy in Britain: The politics and organisation of the National Health Service* (5th edn), Basingstoke: Macmillan.

Help the Aged (2002) *Age discrimination in public policy: A review of the evidence*, London: Help the Aged.

Heywood, N., Lush, D. and Massey, A. (2001) *Heywood and Massey: Court of Protection practice* (13th edn), London: Sweet and Maxwell.

Higgs, P. (1997) 'Citizenship theory and old age: from social rights to surveillance', in A. Jamieson, S. Harper and C. Victor (eds) *Critical approaches to ageing and later life*, Buckingham: Open University Press.

Hockey, J. and James, A. (2003) *Social identities across the life course*, Basingstoke: Palgrave.

House of Commons Health Committee (2004) *Palliative care*, London: The Stationery Office.

Innes, A., Macpherson, S. and McCabe, L. (2006) *Promoting person-care at the front-line*, York: Joseph Rowntree Foundation.

Jamieson, A., Victor, C. and Harper, S. (1997) *Critical approaches to ageing and later life*, Buckingham, Open University Press.

Kennedy, I. (2001) *Learning from Bristol: The report of the Public Inquiry into Children's Heart Surgery at the Bristol Royal Infirmary 1984-1995*, Cm 5207, Bristol: Bristol Royal Infirmary Inquiry.

King's Fund (2002) *Developing intermediate care: A guide for health and social service professionals*, London: King's Fund.

Laing & Buisson (2003) *Long term care: Value of the care market* (www.laingbuisson.co.uk).

Law Commission (1995) *Mental incapacity report no 231*, London: Law Commission.

Law Society (1999) *Guide to the professional conduct of solicitors* (8th edn), London: Law Society.

Letts, P. (1998) *Managing other people's money*, London: Age Concern.

Luce, P. (2003) *The fundamental review of death certification and investigation*, Norwich: The Stationery Office.

Lush, D. and Cretney, S. (2001) *Cretney and Lush on enduring powers of attorney* (5th edn), Bristol: Jordans.

Lymbery, M. (1998) 'Care management and professional autonomy: the impact of community care legislation on social work with older people', *British Journal of Social Work*, vol 28, no 6, pp 863-78.

Lymbery, M. (2005) *Social work with older people: Context, policy and practice*, London: Sage Publications.

McCreadie, C. (1996) *Elder abuse: Update on research*, London: Age Concern Institute of Gerontology.

McDonald, A. (1997) *Challenging local authority decisions*, Birmingham: Venture Press.

McDonald, A. (2006) *Understanding community care: A guide for social workers* (2nd edn), Basingstoke: Palgrave.

McDonald, A. and Taylor, M. (1995) *The law and elderly people*, London: Sweet and Maxwell.

Mitchell, E. (2005) 'Community care law update', *New Law Journal*, vol 155, no 7201, 18 November.

Mitchell, E. (2006) 'Community care update', *New Law Journal*, vol 156, pp 838-9.

Montgomery, J. (2003) *Health care law* (2nd edn), Oxford: Oxford University Press.

NPSA (National Patient Safety Agency) (2005) *Being open*, London: NPSA.

Norman, A. (1985) *Triple jeopardy: Growing old in a second homeland*, London: Centre for Policy in Ageing.

ODPM (Office of the Deputy Prime Minister) (2002) *Code of guidance on homelessness*, London: ODPM.

ODPM (2005) *Guidance on contracting for services in the light of the Human Rights Act 1998*, London: ODPM.

Office of Fair Trading (2003) *A guide on unfair contract terms in care homes contracts: A guide for professional advisers*, London: Office of Fair Trading.

Oldman, C. (2000) *Blurring the boundaries: A fresh look at housing and care provision for older people*, Brighton: Pavilion.

Peace, S., Kellaher, L. and Willcocks, D. (1997) *Re-evaluating residential care*, Buckingham: Open University Press.

Phillips, J., Bernard, M. and Chittenden, M. (2002) *Juggling work and care: The experience of working carers of older adults*, York: Joseph Rowntree Foundation.

Postle, K. (2001) 'The social work side is disappearing: I guess it started with us called care managers', *Practice*, vol 13, no 1, pp 13–26.

Postle, K. (2002) 'Working "between the idea and the reality": ambiguities and tensions in care managers' work', *British Journal of Social Work*, vol 32, no 3, pp 335-51.

Preston-Shoot, M. (2000) 'What if? Using the law to uphold practice values and standards', *Practice*, vol 12, no 4, pp 49-63.

Preston-Shoot, M. and Wigley, V. (2002) 'Closing the circle: social workers' responses to multi-agency procedures on older age abuse', *British Journal of Social Work*, vol 32, pp 299-320.

Priestley, M, and Rabiee (2001) *Building bridges: Disability and old age*, (www.leeds.ac.uk/disability-studies/projects/olderpeople/bridgesreport.pdf).

Richards, S. (2000) 'Bridging the divide: elders and the assessment process', *British Journal of Social Work*, vol 30, pp 37-49.

Richardson, G. (1999) *Proposals by the Mental Health Act Review Expert Committee*, London: DH

Ridout, P. (2003) *Care standards: A practical guide*, Bristol: Jordans.

Roberts, E. (2000) *Age discrimination in health and social care*, London: King's Fund.

Royal College of Physicians (2003) *The vegetative state: Guidance on diagnosis and management*, London: Royal College of Physicians.

Royal Commission on Long-term Care (1999) *With respect to old age: Long-term care: Rights and responsibilities*, London: The Stationery Office.

Schwer, B. (2001) 'Human rights and social services', in L.-A. Cull and J. Roche (eds) *The law and social work: Contemporary issues for practice*, Basingstoke: Palgrave.

SCIE (Social Care Institute for Excellence) (2006) *Assessing the mental health needs of older people*, London: SCIE.

SEU (Social Exclusion Unit) (2006) *A sure start to later life: Ending inequalities for older people*, London: SEU.

Smale, G. and Tuson, G. with Biehal, N. and Marsh, P. (1993) *Empowerment, assessment: Care management and the skilled worker*, London: NISW/HMSO.

Stainton, T. (2002) 'Taking rights structurally: Disability rights and social worker responses to direct payments', *British Journal of Social Work*, vol 32, pp 751-63.

Stalker, K. (2003) *Reconceptualising work with 'carers': New directions for policy and practice*, London: Jessica Kingsley.

Thompson, N. (1995) *Age and dignity: Working with older people*, London: Arena.

TOPSS (Training Organisation for the Personal Social Services) (2001) *National occupational standards for social care workers*, London: TOPSS.

Walker, A. (2005) *Understanding quality of life in old age*, Buckingham: Open University Press.

Wanless, D. (2006) *Securing good care for older people: Taking a long-term view*, London: King's Fund.

Watson, J. and Woolf, M. (2003) *Human Rights Act toolkit*, London: Legal Action Group.

West, S. (2006) *Your rights: A guide to money benefits for older people*, London, Age Concern.

Willcocks, D., Kellaher, L. and Peace, S. (1987) *Private lives in public places*, London: Tavistock.

Index

A

abuse 37–8
  compulsory removal from home 41–2
  legal responses 39–41
  No secrets 38–9
  policy developments 38
  resolving disputes 42–3
Action on Elder Abuse 38
admission for assessment 78
admission for treatment 78–9
admission of mentally incapacitated
  patients 79–80
adult placement schemes 19
advance directives 67, 68–9
aftercare services 19–20, 83–5
Age Concern 67, 103, 121
ageism 6–7
Anti-Social Behaviour Orders 39–40
appointeeship 111, 112
Arksey, H. 36
assessment 9–11
  carers 34–5
  directions 12
  disabled people 20, 21–2
  mental health 74–5, 78
  in practice 14
  Single Assessment Process 12–13
Assessment of mental capacity (BMA and
  Law Society) 111
Assisted Dying for the Terminally Ill Bill
  73
Association of Directors of Social
  Services (ADSS) 39
assured shorthold tenancies 92
assured tenancies 92
asylum seekers, residential care 17, 97–8
Attendance Allowance 98, 125, 127–9,
  130, 131, 133
Audit Commission
  Fully equipped 23–4
  mental health services 73
  NSF for older people 58–9

B

bed blocking 63–4
benefits *see* social security benefits
bereavement benefits 126
best interest decisions 69–70
Blue Badges 128
boarding out services 19

breach of statutory duty 47–8
British Bankers' Association (BBA) 118
British Institute of Human Rights 50
British Medical Association
  Assessment of mental capacity 111
  DNR decisions 70–1

C

Capital Gains Tax 118, 143
care homes, definition 105
Care Management and assessment:
  Practitioners' guide (DH) 4, 10, 11, 28
care plan 26–7
  commissioning services 28–9
  targeting resources 29
  unmet needs 29
Care Programme Approach (CPA) 19,
  74–5
Care Standards Tribunal 108
carers 33–4
  assessments 34–5
  Carers Allowance 129–30
  pensions 123
  rights 36
  services 36–7
  undue influence 119–20
Carers Allowance 129–30
Carers' Grants 37
Centre for Policy on Ageing 13
Charging for Residential
  Accommodation Guide (CRAG) 133
Child Poverty Action Group 123
Child Tax Credit 123, 124
Clark, H. 33
Code of guidance on homelessness (DCLG)
  95
cold weather payments 124–5
Commission for Equality and Human
  Rights 121
Commission for Social Care Inspection
  v, 104
  complaints 45
  hospital discharge 64
  inspections 108
  NSF for older people 58–9
  registration of care homes 107
community care assessment directions, The
  (DH) 3–4, 12
community care grants 125

Community care in the next decade and beyond (DH) 4, 34
community care services v, 5, 9, 16–20
  abuse 37–43
  aftercare 83–5
  assessment 9–14
  care plan 26–9
  carers' assessments and carers' services 33–7
  challenging decisions 43–50
  charges 131–2
  direct payments 30–3
  disability services 20–6
  and health care services 56–7
  reviews 29–30
  service provision 14–20
complaints
  community care services 43–50
  health care 87–8
confidentiality 13–14
consumerism 5, 9
continuing NHS care 46, 60–2
cooking test 127
coroners 138–40
Council for the Regulation of Healthcare Professionals 55
Council Tax Benefit 125, 129, 130–1
Court of Protection 67, 82, 111, 114
  receivership 115–18
CSCI *see* Commission for Social Care Inspection

D

Dawson, C. 33
day services 19
death 137
  coroners 138–40
  distribution of estate 140–2
  funeral arrangements 137–8
  taxation 143–4
  see also end of life issues
delayed discharges 63–4
Department for Constitutional Affairs (DCA) 138
Department for Work and Pensions
  appointeeship 112
  benefits 123
  funerals 138
  residential care 96
  Social Fund 125
Department of Health (DH)
  Care Programme Approach 74
  CI (95)12 34

Circular 17/96 24
Circular 19/71 17
Discharge from hospital 64
HSC 1998/048 103
LAC (93)7 96–7
LAC (93)10 17, 19
LAC (98)19 98
LAC (2001)1 59
LAC (2001)32 131
LAC (2003)14 59
LAC (2006)12 133
LASSL (97)13 23
The right to complain 43
Developing services for carers and families of people with mental illness (DH) 35
direct payments 30–2, 132
  continuing NHS care services 46
  research findings 33
  support services 32
Disability Alliance 123
Disability and Carers Service 123
Disability Living Allowance 98, 123, 125, 127–9, 130, 131–2, 133
disability services 14, 17, 18, 20–2
  equipment and adaptations 23–6
  service list 22–3
Disabled Facilities Grants 24
Discharge from hospital (DH) 64
discrimination 6–7
  direct payments 33
  employment 120–1
DNR (do not resuscitate) decisions 70–1
domiciliary services 18

E

elders *see* older people
Employment and Support Allowance 127
Employment Directive 2000/78 7, 120
employment rights 120–1
Empowerment Orders 116–17
end of life issues 70
  palliative care 65
  permanent vegetative state 71–2
  resuscitation 70–1
  right to die 72–3
  withdrawal of treatment 71
  see also death
enduring power of attorney (EPA) 32, 40, 113–14, 115
equipment 24
equity release schemes 118–19
Essex County Council 30

European Economic Community
  Directive 97/7 122

F

Fair access to care services (DH) 10, 11, 15,
  27, 28, 29, 123
family provision 142-3
financial management v, 40, 111
  appointeeship 112
  charging for non-residential services
    131-2
  employment rights 120-1
  equity release schemes 118-19
  lifetime gifts 118
  paying for residential care 133-4
  pensions 121-3
  powers of attorney 112-15
  social security benefits 123-31
  undue influence 119-20
First General Order 116
freedom of information 14
Fully equipped (Audit Commission) 23-4
funerals
  arrangements 137-8
  benefits 124

G

General Social Care Council 87
Gloucestershire 23
GPs (general practitioners) 55
guardianship 81-2

H

health care v, 53-4
  challenging decisions 46, 87-8
  consent to treatment 66
  end of life issues 70-3
  hospital discharge 63-5
  intermediate care 59
  joint working 14, 56-7
  legal basis of NHS care 54-5
  mental health 73-86
  mental incapacity 66-70
  NHS continuing care 46, 60-2
  NHS treatment abroad 62-3
  NSF for older people 57-9
  palliative care 65
  responsibility for community health
    care 55-6
Healthcare Commission
  annual audit 55
  NSF for older people 58-9
  reviews of complaints 88

Higgs, P. 9
HM Revenue & Customs 123
home care services 18
Home Repairs Assistance 24
homelessness 94-6
hospital discharge 63-5
House of Commons Health Committee
  65
housing 91
  adaptations 24-6
  assessment 14
  homelessness 94-6
  Housing Benefit and Council Tax
    Benefit 130-1
  owner-occupation 91
  supported housing 93-4
  tenancies in the public and private
    sector 92-3
Housing Benefit 93, 94, 125, 129, 130-1

I

Incapacity Benefit 126-7
Income Support 124, 127, 129, 130, 131
individual budgets 33
Inheritance Tax 118, 143-4
inquests 139-40
inter-agency working 14, 56-7
intermediate care 59
Invalidity Benefit 126

J

Jobcentre Plus 123
Jobseeker's Allowance 122, 124, 125
joint working 14, 56-7
judicial review 49-50

K

King's Fund 59

L

lasting powers of attorney 67, 69, 112,
  113, 114-15
Law Commission 38, 42, 66
Law Society 111
lawyers 2-3
lifetime gifts 118
Living well in later life (Audit Commission)
  58-9
Living Wills 67, 68-9
local authorities
  actions for breach of statutory duty
    47-8
  actions in negligence 48-9

aftercare 83–5
assessment 8–14
care plan 26–9
community care services charges 131–2
community care services provision
    14–20
complaints procedures 43–4
default powers 46–7
direct payments 30–3
disability services 20–6
funerals 137
guardianship 82
and homelessness 94–6
hospital discharge 63–4
monitoring officers 47
ombudsman 45–6
residential care 98–100, 101–3, 104,
    133–4
reviews of services 29–30
sources of law 3–4

M

meals services 19
men
    bereavement benefits 126
    pensions 122
mental disorder, definition 77–8
mental health 73–4
    admission for assessment 78
    admission of mentally incapacitated
        patients 79–80
    admission for treatment 78–9
    aftercare duties 19–20, 83–5
    Care Programme Approach 74–5
    carers 35
    complex cases funding 80–1
    guardianship 81–2
    mental disorder 77–8
    Mental Health Act 1983 75–6
    Mental Health Act 1983 reform 85–6
    mental health review tribunals 82–3
    nearest relative 76–7
    powers of entry and powers of
        detection 79
mental health review tribunals 82–3
mental incapacity 66–8
    admission on mental health grounds
        79–80
    advance directives 68–9
    best interest decisions 69–70
    lasting power of attorney 69
Merton London Borough Council 100
monitoring officers 47

N

National Asylum Support Service
    (NASS) 97–8
National Care Standards Commission
    (NCSC) 104
National Health Service (NHS)
    aids and equipment 24
    complaints procedures 88
    continuing care 60–2
    funerals 137
    inter-agency working 53
    legal basis of care 3, 54–5
    ombudsman 45, 46
    palliative care 65
    reorganisation v
    treatment abroad 62–3
    see also health care
*National Health Service end of life care
    programme, The* (DH) 65
National Health Service Litigation
    Authority 88
National Insurance Retirement Pension
    112
*National occupational standards for social
    workers* (TOPSS) 7–8
National Patient Safety Agency 87–8
National Pensions Saving Scheme 122
National service framework for mental
    health 35
National service framework for older people
    (DH) v, 10, 29, 56–9
national service frameworks (NSFs) 53
nearest relative 76–7
negligence 40, 48–9, 87, 102
*Next steps in implementing the national
    service framework for older people* (DH)
    58
NICE (National Institute for Clinical
    Excellence) 55
No secrets (DH) 38–9
nursing care 55–6

O

Office of Fair Trading 102
Office of the Public Guardian 115
older people 1, 147–8
    absence of legal framework 1–2
    abuse 37–43
    discrimination 6–7
    social policy context 5–6
ombudsmen 45–6, 88, 100
owner-occupation 91

P

palliative care 65
Part III accommodation 16-17
Patient Advice and Liaison Service
    (PALS) 88
Pension Credit v, 122, 123-4, 125, 126,
    131, 134
  housing costs 91, 130
  severe disability element 129
Pension Service 123
pensions 6
  proposed changes 122-3
  state pensions 121-2
permanent vegetative state 71-2
Phillips, J. 36
Pointon Case 46, 60
police, powers of entry and detention 79
power of attorney 111
  financial management 112-15
  see also enduring power of attorney;
    lasting power of attorney
powers of detention 79
powers of entry 79
Practitioners' guide (NHS and Community
    Care Act) (DH) 4, 10, 11, 28
*Practitioners' guide to carers assessment under
    the Carers and Disabled Children Act
    2000* (DH) 35
Preston-Shoot, M. 39
Primary Health Care Need Approach 61
Public Guardianship Office 114, 115

R

receivership 40, 111, 115-18
Registered Nursing Care Contribution
    (RNCC) 56, 62
regulated tenancies 92
Renovations Grants 24
residential care 16-17, 96-7
  choice in accommodation 100-1
  closure of care homes 102-3
  conditions of registration 106
  contractural issues 101-2
  definition of registered care homes 105
  Disability Living Allowance and
    Attendance Allowance 129
  meaning of residential accommodation
    97
  need for care and attention 97-100
  paying for 133-4
  range of people required to register
    105-6
  regulation 104-5

regulations and national minimum
    standards 106-8
  reviews 30
  sanctions and appeals 108
resuscitation 70-1
Richardson Committee 85
Ridout, P. 104, 106
Right to Buy 92-3
right to die 72-3
Royal College of Physicians, permanent
    vegetative state 71, 72
Royal Commission on Long-term Care
    91

S

Scotland, free personal care 91
sectioning 76-7
Severe Disablement Allowance 124
sheltered housing 93-4
Shipman Inquiry 139
Sickness Benefit 126
Single Assessment Process (SAP) 12-13,
    27, 56-7, 74
Social Care Institute for Excellence
    (SCIE) 74, 78
Social Fund 124-5
social security benefits 6, 123, 125-6
  appointeeship 112
  bereavement benefits 126
  Carers Allowance 129-30
  Disability Living Allowance and
    Attendance Allowance 127-9
  Housing Benefit and Council Tax
    Benefit 130-1
  Incapacity Benefit 126-7
  Income Support 124
  Pension Credit 123-4
  Social Fund 124-5
social work services 17-18
social workers
  liability 48
  powers of entry 79
  roles 2-3, 7-8
Stainton, T. 33
Stalker, K. 35
state pensions 121-3
supported housing 93-4
Supporting People 93, 94, 130

T

taxation 143-4
television licences 126
tenancies 92-3
travel 126

U

undue influence 119-20
unmet needs 29
user-controlled trusts 132

W

Wanless report 91
Warm Front grants 125-6
Widowed Parent's Allowance 126
Wigley, V. 39
winter fuel payments 125
withdrawal of treatment 71
women
  bereavement benefits 126
  pensions 122
Working Tax Credit 123

Y

York City Council 84
young carers 34

Available from BASW/The Policy Press

Social work and people with dementia
Partnerships, practice and persistence
Mary Marshall and **Margaret-Anne Tibbs**

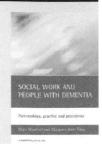

Current community care policies and increasing numbers of older people needing assistance mean that all social workers must be up-to-date in their knowledge, skills and attitudes towards people with dementia and their carers. This book, written by experienced social workers, provides guidance on best practice in a readable and jargon-free style.

This book is essential reading for social work and social care students, social workers undertaking CPD, and social and care workers transferring to dementia care from other fields.

PB £17.99 US$29.95 **ISBN-10** 1 86134 702 2 **ISBN-13** 978 1 86134 702 2
HB £55.00 US$75.00 **ISBN-10** 1 86134 703 0 **ISBN-13** 978 1 86134 703 9
234 x 156mm 256 pages tbc November 2006

Working in group care
Social work and social care in residential and day care settings
(Revised Second Edition)
Adrian Ward

This book illustrates how best practice can be achieved in residential and care settings through the focused and engaged work of individuals and teams who are well supported and managed. Recognising the challenging and complex nature of group care, detailed attention is paid to the value of everyday practice and its underlying principles.

This second edition book brings together theory, practice and research findings from across the whole field of group care for all user-groups, including health, education and probation settings as well as social work and social care.

PB £17.99 US$29.95 **ISBN-10** 1 86134 706 5 **ISBN-13** 978 1 86134 706 0
HB £55.00 US$75.00 **ISBN-10** 1 86134 707 3 **ISBN-13** 978 1 86134 707 7
234 x 156mm 232 pages tbc November 2006

What is professional social work?
(Revised Second Edition)
Malcolm Payne

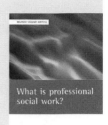

"The author is outstanding in his ability to write fluently, compassionately and with a depth of understanding informed by unsurpassed knowledge of his field. What is professional social work? fills a notable gap in the literature, namely by providing an accessible entry into debates about the nature and standing of social work as a profession."
Robert Adams, Professor of Social Work, School of Health and Social Care, University of Teeside, UK

What is Professional Social Work? is a now classic analysis of social work as a discourse between three aspects of practice: social order, therapeutic and transformational perspectives. It enables social workers to analyse and value the role of social work in present-day multiprofessional social care.

This new edition will stimulate social workers, students and policy-makers in social care to think again about the valuable role social work plays in society.

PB £16.99 US$29.95 **ISBN-10** 1 86134 704 9 **ISBN-13** 978 1 86134 704 6
HB £55.00 US$80.00 **ISBN-10** 1 86134 705 7 **ISBN-13** 978 1 86134 705 3
234 x 156mm 232 pages July 2006

To order copies of this publication or any other Policy Press titles please visit **www.policypress.org.uk** or contact:

In the UK and Europe:
Marston Book Services, PO Box 269,
Abingdon, Oxon, OX14 4YN, UK
Tel: +44 (0)1235 465500
Fax: +44 (0)1235 465556
Email: direct.orders@marston.co.uk

In the USA and Canada:
ISBS, 920 NE 58th Street,
Suite 300, Portland, OR
97213-3786, USA
Tel: +1 800 944 6190
(toll free)
Fax: +1 503 280 8832
Email: info@isbs.com

**In Australia and
New Zealand:**
DA Information Services,
648 Whitehorse Road Mitcham,
Victoria 3132, Australia
Tel: +61 (3) 9210 7777
Fax: +61 (3) 9210 7788
E-mail: service@dadirect.com.au